Clinical Skills for Pharmacists

A PATIENT-FOCUSED APPROACH

Clinical Skills
for Pharmacists

A PATIENT-FOCUSED APPROACH

KAREN J. TIETZE, PharmD
Associate Professor of Clinical Pharmacy
Philadelphia College of Pharmacy and Science
Philadelphia, Pennsylvania

with 36 illustrations

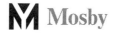

St. Louis Baltimore Boston Carlsbad Chicago Minneapolis New York Philadelphia Portland
London Milan Sydney Tokyo Toronto

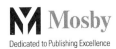

Dedicated to Publishing Excellence

A Times Mirror
Company

Vice President and Publisher: Don Ladig
Editor: Jennifer Roche
Developmental Editor: Sandra J. Parker/Laura MacAdam
Project Manager: Linda McKinley
Production Editor: Jennifer Furey
Designer: Renée Duenow
Manufacturing Supervisor: Don Carlisle

Printed in the United States of America

Composition by Clarinda Co.
Lithography by Top Graphics, Inc.
Printing/binding by Maple Vail Book Manufacturing Co.

Mosby–Year Book, Inc.
11830 Westline Industrial Drive
St. Louis, Missouri 63146.

Library of Congress Cataloging in Publication Data
Tietze, Karen J.
    Clinical skills for pharmacists: a patient-focused approach /
Karen J. Tietze.
        p.   cm.
    Includes bibliographical references and index.
    ISBN 0-8016-6484-5
    1. Pharmacy.   2. Pharmacy—Practice.   3. Communication in
pharmacy.   I. Title.
    [DNLM: 1. Pharmaceutical Services.   2. Pharmacy—methods.   QV 737
T564c   1997]
RS91.T54   1997
615'.1—dc21
DNLM/DLC
for Library of Congress   97-11635
                                                                 CIP

97 98 99 00 01/9 8 7 6 5 4 3 2 1

To my students

Preface

THIS book grew out of my desire to teach patient-focused skills, such as how to present a patient case, obtain a medication history, and monitor a therapeutic regimen, to pharmacy students prior to their clerkships. As a young faculty member, I was frustrated by the lack of resources and by teaching these skills during clerkship. I began to suspect that many patient-focused skills could be more efficiently taught in a classroom setting and did not require interactions with "real" patients. I also began to suspect that students could benefit by learning these skills very early in their education. It was at about this time that the profession embraced the philosophy of pharmaceutical care and began widespread implementation of 6-year Doctor of Pharmacy degree programs and Doctor of Pharmacy degree programs for licensed pharmacists, all of which greatly increased the demand for these skills. Fortunately I was able to develop this book as I developed first an elective skills course and then required skills courses for our baccalaureate, 6-year Doctor of Pharmacy, and flexible Doctor of Pharmacy programs. These experiences were invaluable in shaping the content and character of the book.

This textbook is intended to be used as a tool for teaching the skills necessary for the provision of pharmaceutical care. Pharmacy students learning these skills in the classroom setting or while on clerkship as well as pharmacists who desire to become more involved in the provision of pharmaceutical care should benefit by reading and studying the book. It is also the first book that brings together all the information on communication skills, physical assessment skills, laboratory and diagnostic tests, the patient case presentation, therapeutic planning and monitoring skills, drug information skills, and ethics. As such, it should serve as a useful reference for all pharmacists. It was not my intent to create a clerkship manual, a comprehensive physical assessment textbook, or a comprehensive ethics textbook. Rather, my hope is that this textbook will complement the excellent resources already available on these topics.

Organization of the book deliberately places fundamental skills (communication skills, physical assessment skills, and laboratory and diagnostic information) prior to the chapters on the patient case presentation, therapeutic planning, and monitoring. Numerous patient case examples are used throughout the book. Each skill is designed to build on prior skills; development of each skill depends on integration and application of previous skills. I have tried to provide an obvious structure and organizational process, especially for the development of the skills necessary for the selection and monitoring of patient-specific therapeutic regimens. As with all first editions, this book remains a work in progress. All suggestions are welcomed.

Karen J. Tietze

Acknowledgments

IT is impossible to individually acknowledge all those who contributed to the development of this book. I thank the hundreds of students who taught me what works and what doesn't work when learning these skills. I also thank my colleagues at the Philadelphia College of Pharmacy and Science whose moral support throughout this process was invaluable.

Special thanks to the following individuals who provided detailed reviews of one or more chapters:

Jerry L. Bauman, PharmD, *Professor, College of Pharmacy, University of Illinois at Chicago*
Janice A. Gaska, PharmD, *Manager, Medical Communications, Zeneca Pharmaceuticals*
Arthur I. Jacknowitz, PharmD, *Professor, College of Pharmacy, West Virginia University*
Paul L. Ranelli, PhD, *Associate Professor, School of Pharmacy, University of Wyoming*
Timothy H. Self, PharmD, *Professor, College of Pharmacy, University of Tennessee*

I am especially indebted to Dr. Janice Gaska. Our original plan was to coauthor the book. We spent countless hours planning and outlining the book before she left PCPS. The book reflects both of our philosophies and is much better than I could have created on my own.

I am also indebted to Sandra Parker, Developmental Editor, Laura MacAdam, Developmental Editor, Jennifer Roche, Acquisitions Editor, and Jennifer Furey, Production Editor, Mosby–Year Book, Inc. Their guidance was invaluable. Their enthusiasm was a great motivation.

Finally, thanks to my family for their support and understanding of what it takes to get this type of project completed.

Karen J. Tietze

Contents

Clinical Skills for Pharmacists

A PATIENT-FOCUSED APPROACH

C H A P T E R   1

Introduction: The Practice
of Clinical Pharmacy

LEARNING OBJECTIVES

1 Define pharmaceutical care and identify the four outcomes that improve a patient's quality of life.
2 List the knowledge and skills needed for patient-focused pharmacy practice.
3 State the eligibility requirements for board certification and identify the areas available for certification.
4 Differentiate between residencies and fellowships in terms of definition, length of training, and mechanisms for credentialing.
5 Identify and differentiate among the various types of health care settings and environments.
6 State the purpose of the medical team and identify the roles and responsibilities of each member.
7 Identify and describe unresolved health care system issues.

THE emphasis in pharmacy practice is evolving away from managing the distribution of drug products toward providing patient-focused (also known as *patient-centered*) services. To be successful, pharmacists must understand and speak the language of the health care system and function in a system that to the uninitiated is foreign and excessively complex. The variety of providers, rapidly evolving types of health care delivery systems, and complexities of relationships among the various health care professionals working within the health care system also add confusion. This chapter demystifies the health care system by describing patient-focused pharmacy practice and the clinical environment in which patient-focused pharmacists function.

PATIENT-FOCUSED PHARMACY PRACTICE

The term *clinical pharmacy* has historically been used to describe patient-oriented rather than product-oriented pharmacy practice. Patient-focused pharmacy practice, which focuses on patient care rather than management of drug products, requires the integration of a broad range of data and skills (Figure 1-1). Historically, the term *clinical pharmacist* was used to describe a pharmacist whose primary job was to interact with the health care team, interview and assess patients, make specific therapeutic recommendations, monitor patient response to drug therapy, and provide drug information. Clinical pharmacists, working primarily in acute care settings, were viewed as "drug experts"; other pharmacists could occasionally use "clinical" skills, but their practices remained focused on product management. The profession of pharmacy has evolved to the point that many pharmacists find the

1

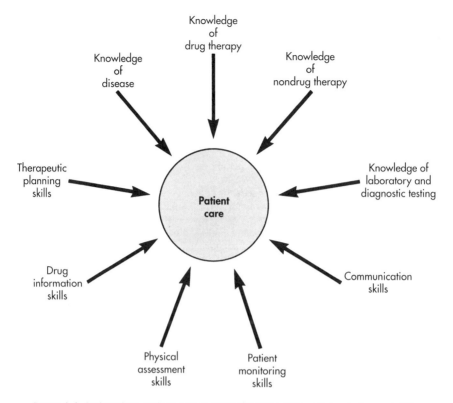

FIGURE 1-1 *Patient Care.* Patient care requires the integration of knowledge and skills.

term *clinical pharmacy* redundant; they emphasize that the practice of pharmacy requires all pharmacists to provide patient-focused services.

The term *pharmaceutical care* is used to describe the broad-based, patient-focused responsibilities of pharmacists. Hepler and Strand define pharmaceutical care as the "responsible provision of drug therapy for the purpose of achieving definite outcomes that improve a patient's quality of life."[1] The four outcomes they identified include the following:

1. Cure of disease
2. Elimination or reduction of symptoms
3. Arrest or slowing of a disease process
4. Prevention of disease or symptoms

The philosophy of pharmaceutical care embodies the concept that pharmacists work with the patient and the health care team in determining and providing the most appropriate pharmacotherapy for the patient.

Patient-focused pharmacy practice requires an expert knowledge of therapeutics, a good understanding of disease processes, and a knowledge of drug products. In addition, patient-focused pharmacy practice requires strong communication skills, drug monitoring skills, provision of drug information, therapeutic planning skills, and the ability to assess and interpret physical assessment findings.

Box 1-1	*Patient-Focused Practice Areas*
Ambulatory care	Nephrology
Critical care	Obstetrics and gynecology
Drug information	Pulmonary disease
Geriatrics and long-term care	Psychiatry
Internal medicine and subspecialties	Rheumatology
Cardiology	Nuclear pharmacy
Endocrinology	Nutrition
Gastroenterology	Pediatrics
Infectious disease	Pharmacokinetics
Neurology	Surgery

Sites and Types of Practice

Patient-focused pharmacy practice can be performed anywhere patients are treated, including teaching and community hospitals, outpatient clinics, community pharmacies, long-term care facilities, and patients' homes. Some pharmacists are full-time practitioners in specialty practice areas such as pediatrics, critical care, nutrition, and cardiology; these areas are similar to traditional medical specialty or subspecialty areas. Other practice areas, including drug information and pharmacokinetics, are unique to pharmacy (Box 1-1).

Patient-focused pharmacists work closely with physicians and other health care professionals to provide optimal patient care. Some pharmacists in traditional product-centered practice settings use clinical pharmacy skills in a limited capacity, such as when they obtain a medication history or recommend specific nonprescription drug therapy. Other pharmacists have no traditional product-centered responsibilities and instead provide full-time pharmaceutical care. Regardless of the setting and the degree to which patient-focused skills are used, pharmaceutical care is an integral part of the practice of pharmacy.

The only requirement for the provision of patient-focused services is an adequate background and training. Pharmacists with Bachelor of Science in Pharmacy degrees or Doctor of Pharmacy degrees provide patient-focused services. The largest difference between the two educational programs is that Doctor of Pharmacy programs provide more intensive experience and training in the data and skills necessary for patient-focused practice than do traditional 5-year baccalaureate programs. Postgraduate training programs provide the pharmacist with even more intensive supervised experience and training.

Certification

Board certification is evolving to recognize that pharmacists have specific knowledge and skills. Board certification is acquired in addition to state and federal licensure requirements. Some employers require board certification for certain jobs such as nutrition support and clinical coordinator positions; other employers reward board certification with career advancement and salary differentials. The Board of Pharmaceutical Specialties (BPS), created in 1976 by the American Pharmaceutical Association, is responsible for setting standards for certification and recertification and administering certification and recertification processes. Certification by written examination is available in pharmacotherapy, nutrition, nuclear pharmacy, and psychiatric pharmacy practice; certification of other areas is under

Box 1-2	*Postgraduate Pharmacy Residency Programs*	
Administration	Family medicine	Nutrition
Ambulatory care	Gastroenterology	Oncology
Cardiology	General medicine	Pediatrics
Community pharmacy	Geriatrics	Pharmacokinetics
Critical care	Hospital pharmacy	Pharmacotherapy
Dermatology	Infectious disease	Psychiatry
Drug information	Nephrology	Toxicology

consideration. Pharmacists with advanced education (Doctor of Pharmacy degrees) and training or equivalent experience are eligible for certification. The BPS requires that board-certified pharmacists complete periodic recredentialing requirements, which typically consist of completion of specified types of continuing education and reexamination. Board-certified pharmacists are entitled to denote the accomplishment in their title (e.g., Board-Certified Pharmacotherapy Specialist [BCPS], Board-Certified Nutrition Support Pharmacist [BCNSP], Board-Certified Nuclear Pharmacist [BCNP], Board-Certified Psychiatric Pharmacist [BCPP]).

Postgraduate Training

Pharmacy graduates may obtain additional experience, knowledge, and skills by participating in a variety of residency and fellowship postgraduate training programs. Although most residency and fellowship programs require candidates to have either entry-level or postbaccalaureate Doctor of Pharmacy degrees, some general and administrative residency programs are available for 5-year baccalaureate pharmacy graduates.

A *residency* is defined as an "organized, directed, postgraduate training program in a defined area of pharmacy practice."[2] Residencies provide pharmacists 1- to 2-year supervised experiences in practice and management activities. Residencies may be general, providing broad-based experiences, or specialized in such focused areas as ambulatory care, critical care, drug information, and pharmacokinetics (Box 1-2). Residents generally gain experience providing drug information, pharmacokinetics, and a variety of other inpatient and outpatient pharmacy services. In the past, most residencies were based in hospitals; however, both interest in and the availability of community pharmacy-based, patient-focused residencies have been growing. The American Society of Health-System Pharmacists (ASHP) accredits residency programs.

A pharmacy fellowship is a highly individualized program designed to prepare the pharmacist to become an independent researcher.[2] Applicants for fellowships are expected to have completed Doctor of Pharmacy and residency programs or to have equivalent experience. Fellowships provide pharmacists with 1 to 3 years of supervised research experience in highly focused areas such as pharmacokinetics and pharmacodynamics, oncology, nephrology, infectious disease, critical care, and pediatrics (Box 1-3). Fellows spend approximately 80% of their time in research-related activities. Currently no mechanism for accreditation of fellowship programs is available. However, the American College of Clinical Pharmacy (ACCP) Fellowship Review Committee conducts a voluntary peer review program; 14 fellowship programs were recognized in 1996 as meeting ACCP guidelines for research training programs.

Box 1-3	*Postgraduate Pharmacy Fellowship Training Programs*	
Ambulatory care	Family medicine	Oncology
Analgesia	Gastroenterology	Pediatrics
Cardiology	General medicine	Pharmacodynamics
Critical care	Geriatrics	Pharmacokinetics
Dermatology	Infectious disease	Psychiatry
Drug development	Nephrology	Pulmonary disease
Drug information	Neurology	Rheumatology
Drug metabolism	Nutrition	

Information regarding residency and fellowship programs can be obtained from national directories. The ASHP publishes a directory of ASHP-accredited residency programs, and the ACCP publishes a directory of residency and fellowship programs offered by members of the ACCP. Both directories are updated annually.

THE CLINICAL ENVIRONMENT

Health care is provided in many different settings (Box 1-4). Outpatient services are available at private physicians' offices, outpatient clinics, day surgery units (also known as *short procedure units*), and emergency rooms. Patients are hospitalized for major surgery, treatment of acute disorders, and diagnostic evaluations and procedures. Long-term care facilities such as nursing homes and rehabilitation centers provide health care for patients who require skilled management of chronic disorders. Home health care services are available for chronically ill or disabled patients.

Physicians provide inpatient and outpatient health care services in individual and group practices. Group practices may consist of associations of specialists (e.g., internal medicine, surgery, family medicine) or several different types of physician specialties (e.g., family medicine, obstetrics and gynecology, cardiology, orthopedics) that provide broad-based medical services to the patient. Although some physicians maintain individual practices, most physicians' practices have changed dramatically in response to the rapid evolution of health care delivery in the 1990s from traditional fee-for-service (FFS) indemnity insurance plans in which patients are free to select any physicians they wish to managed care insurance plans in which patients are restricted to participating physicians. Many different types of alliances have been formed among physicians, health care institutions, and insurers, including physician networks, prepaid group practices, and integrated delivery systems.

Clinics, often affiliated with major medical centers and hospitals, are located in outpatient areas of hospitals and other facilities. Clinics provide outpatient health care for specific patient groups and are often identified by the specific patient population served by the clinic. Common types include hypertension, diabetes, rheumatology, orthopedics, oncology, nephrology, and anticoagulation clinics. Several clinics may use the same outpatient care areas; in this situation the schedule is set to allow each clinic to have a unique weekly or daily schedule (e.g., anticoagulation clinic on Tuesday afternoons, diabetes clinic on Wednesday mornings, hypertension clinic on Friday mornings).

Hospitals are described as public, private, or federal hospitals, depending on the way the hospital is funded. Public hospitals are publicly funded institutions that

---

Box 1-4   *Health Care Settings*

OUTPATIENT	INPATIENT
Clinics	Hospitals
Day surgery units	
Emergency rooms	LONG-TERM CARE FACILITIES
Home health care	Rehabilitation centers
Private offices	Skilled nursing homes

Box 1-5   *Allied Health Care Professionals*

Anesthesiologist's Assistant	Medical Technologist
Cardiovascular Technologist	Occupational Therapist
Cytotechnologist	Ophthalmic Medical Assistant
Diagnostic Medical Sonographer	Perfusionist
Electroencephalographic Technologist	Physician Assistant
Emergency Medical Technician	Radiation Therapy Technologist
Histologic Technician	Radiographer
Medical Assistant	Respiratory Therapist
Medical Illustrator	Respiratory Therapy Technician
Medical Laboratory Technician	Specialist in Blood Bank Technology
Medical Record Administrator	Surgeon's Assistant/Technologist
Medical Record Technician	

---

provide health care services regardless of the ability of the patient to pay or the type of insurance or health coverage of the patient. Some cities and states pay for public hospital services from tax revenues. Private hospitals are privately funded institutions whose services are generally not available, except for emergency care, to patients who are not part of the private group. Federal hospitals are funded by the federal government. The Veterans Administration hospital system, for instance, is an extensive national system of hospitals, clinics, and nursing homes funded by the federal government to provide health care services to American armed forces veterans.

Hospitals may be characterized in other ways. For example, many hospitals, regardless of their funding sources, are affiliated with medical schools. These hospitals, known as *teaching hospitals*, provide training sites for physicians and other health care professionals. Community-based, nonteaching hospitals are sometimes known as *community hospitals*. Some hospitals, recognized for their highly specialized services and large referral patient population, are known as *tertiary hospitals*. Children's hospitals and some oncology hospitals are examples of tertiary hospitals.

Health Care Professionals

Health care professionals include physicians, pharmacists, and nurses. Allied health care professionals, also known as *paramedicals*, provide health care services and perform tasks under the direction of physicians (Box 1-5).

Box 1-6	*Physician Practice Areas*

MEDICAL	**SURGICAL**	**OTHER**
Allergy and immunology	Cardiothoracic	Anesthesiology
Dermatology	Colorectal	Emergency medicine
Family practice	General	Nuclear medicine
General practice	Neurologic	Pathology
Internal medicine	Obstetric and gynecologic	Physical medicine and reha-
Cardiovascular medicine	Ophthalmologic	bilitation
Critical care	Orthopedic	Preventive medicine
Endocrinology	Otorhinolaryngologic	Radiology
Gastroenterology	Plastic	
Hematology	Urologic	
Infectious disease		
Medical oncology		
Nephrology		
Neurology		
Pulmonary disease		
Rheumatology		
Geriatric medicine		
Pediatrics		
Psychiatry		

Physicians, doctors who have medical or osteopathic degrees, are generally considered the leaders of health care teams and have the ultimate responsibility for patient care. Allopathic physicians rely on standard treatment modalities; osteopathic physicians use the additional technique of spine and joint manipulation to treat disease.

Physicians practice medicine in many general and specialty areas (Box 1-6). Family practice physicians, general internal medicine physicians, and pediatric physicians treat patients with a wide variety of diseases. Specialists such as nephrologists and cardiologists treat patients within a narrow spectrum of disease. Many internists (physicians specializing in internal medicine) elect to specialize in one of the many subspecialty areas of internal medicine such as nephrology, cardiology, oncology, pulmonary disease, infectious disease, and neurology. Some confusion regarding certification and specialization may occur because physicians who are not certified are not prohibited from practicing medicine in any specialty or subspecialty they choose.

Physicians are credentialed by national examination and licensed by individual states. Physicians must have degrees from accredited medical schools, receive passing grades on medical licensure examinations (usually the National Board of Medical Examiners examination), and (in most states) complete 1 year of an accredited residency program to become licensed to practice medicine. Relicensure requires completion of continuing medical education requirements. Most physicians obtain 1 or more additional years of supervised experience in residency programs; some complete additional training in highly specialized fellowship programs. The length of the residency program depends on the specialty or subspecialty. For example, internal medicine residencies are typically 3 years in duration; surgical residencies may be 5 to 7 years.

Nurses care for the physical and psychosocial needs of patients and carry out physician-directed orders regarding patient care. Nurses perform many routine tasks for physicians, including patient interviews and examinations, treatment of minor illnesses, and patient education and counseling. Nurses may have Associate Degrees in Nursing (ADNs) obtained from 2-year junior or community colleges, diplomas from 2- to 3-year nursing programs offered by some hospitals and private schools, or Bachelor of Science in Nursing (BSN) degrees from 4-year colleges and universities. Graduates from all three programs are eligible for licensure as registered nurses (RNs); continuing licensure is often contingent on completion of continuing nursing education requirements. Nurse administrators, educators, researchers, clinical specialists, and nurse practitioners usually have master's or doctoral degrees. Nurses may specialize in more than 38 categories based on disease states, patient age, and acuity of illness. Certification is available for some of these specialties. For example, nurses can be certified in critical care and are then entitled to use the designation *Certified Critical Care Registered Nurse (CCRN)* in their titles.

Physician assistants (PAs) perform many routine tasks for physicians such as patient interviews and examinations, treatment of minor illnesses, and patient education and counseling; PAs may prescribe medications in many states. They may have certificates, associate degrees, or master's degrees. Most states require graduates of accredited programs to pass certifying examinations. Those who pass the examination may use the designation *Physician Assistant–Certified (PA–C)*. Continuing licensure is contingent on completion of continuing education requirements; recertification examinations must be passed periodically.

The Health Care Team

The health care team consists of all health care professionals who have responsibility for patient care. The patient is an important member of the health care team. Although all members of the health care team interact directly with the patient, they rarely meet as a group; instead, information and recommendations are exchanged through written documentation. Verbal information exchange and recommendations may occur on a less formal basis.

All members of the health care team contribute their professions' unique knowledge and skills to the care of the patient. Pharmacists are the "drug experts" on the team and are expected to help the team develop, implement, and monitor the therapeutic plan as well as provide drug information and educational services for the patient and team.

Students, regardless of their professions, play a unique role in the health care team. Although they do not yet hold degrees, they represent their professions and are expected to carry out their professional responsibilities; however, students are under the direct supervision of licensed professionals. For example, pharmacy students are expected to provide pharmaceutical care under the direct supervision of a licensed pharmacy preceptor. The amount of autonomy and ability to prospectively influence the decisions of the health care team gradually develop as students gain experience. Although the types of experiences students have varies with the patient care environment, the professional responsibilities remain the same.

The Medical Team

Teaching hospitals are the primary training sites for health care professionals. Health care services in teaching hospitals are organized around medical teams composed of physicians, medical students, and, depending on the hospital, other health care professionals (Box 1-7). The medical team is organized primarily to provide a structured training environment for physicians. Medical teams are responsible for the care of patients located in distinct areas of the hospital (i.e., specific floors) or patients on specific services located throughout the institution. In the latter case the team may provide a consultation service in a medical subspecialty (e.g., infectious disease) or be identified with a specific physician group practice. The medical team functions as a unit, with the division of labor and the responsibility of each member depending on the level of training of that individual. The team is structured so that each team member receives guidance from a practitioner with more experience. In addition, the team is the focus for teaching, group discussions, and group decision-making processes. Physician team members include, in order of seniority, the attending physician, fellows, residents, and medical students.

Attending Physician. The attending physician is the senior physician on the medical team and is usually assigned to a teaching team for 1 month at a time. This designated physician assumes responsibility for all patients assigned to the team, provides guidance and direction to the team regarding patient care, and educates team members about the diagnosis and treatment of specific diseases. The attending physician is in charge of attending rounds, in which patients are presented to the team, examined, and interviewed; the attending physician leads the team through the decision-making process, helps the team make decisions regarding patient care, and evaluates the performance of team members. Patient presentations may take place in a conference room, in the hallway outside of the patient's room, or in the patient's room. The attending physician spends a short portion of the day with the team and is available for consultation (usually by telephone) throughout the rest of the day.

Fellows. Medical fellows are physicians who have completed residency training and have elected to continue their training in a research-oriented program. Fellows work closely with the attending physician and have fewer direct patient care responsibilities than residents. Fellows serve as consultants and teach junior members of the team. Many fellows are responsible for performing specific invasive procedures such as arterial line placement, bronchoscopy, and endoscopy. Research-intensive, multiyear fellowship programs in medical subspecialty areas such as gastroenterology, cardiology, neurology, and pulmonary medicine are available at many major teaching hospitals.

Residents. Medical residents are physicians who have graduated from medical school and are in structured and supervised residency training programs.

Box 1-7	*Medical Team Composition in Teaching Hospitals*

TYPICAL TEAM MEMBERS	OTHER TEAM MEMBERS
Attending physician	Medical ethicist
Senior or junior medical resident	Nurse
Intern	Occupational therapist
Senior medical student	Pharmacist
Junior medical student	Respiratory therapist
	Social worker
	Students (dental, nursing, pharmacy)

Interns. First-year residents (sometimes designated as postgraduate year 1, PGY1, or PG1) are known as *interns.* Internal medicine internships of at least 1 year often are required before the resident moves on to more specialized training in areas such as surgery and psychiatry. The intern year also is the first of several years of training for physicians interested in practicing internal medicine. Interns, who are licensed physicians, have an intensive and extensive year of training, with frequent night call and direct responsibility for the care of a variety of inpatients and outpatients. Interns typically spend 1-month periods gaining experience in a variety of internal medical services such as general medicine, emergency room services, and intensive care services. In addition, interns usually have set clinic hours and see a variety of outpatients over the course of the year.

Second- and third-year residents. Second-year internal medical residents (sometimes designated as postgraduate year 2, PGY2, or PG2) also are known as *junior admitting residents* (JARs). Third-year medical residents (postgraduate year 3, PGY3, or PG3), also known as *senior admitting residents* (SARs), are in the final year of 3-year internal medicine residency programs. Junior and senior medical residents are assigned to medical teams and are placed in charge of the teams. The resident sets the daily team rounding schedule, sets priorities, coordinates the work of the team, supervises the interns, supervises and works closely with the medical students on the team, and consults with the attending physician. Residents have frequent night call and direct responsibility for a variety of inpatients and outpatients.

Chief medical resident. The chief medical resident is a senior medical resident who, in addition to the usual responsibilities of residents, has administrative responsibilities for various aspects of the residency program such as scheduling rotations and vacations and organizing and overseeing seminars and other educational programs. The chief medical resident position is a competitive one; typically one or two residents per year are selected for this position.

Medical Students. Medical students also are members of the medical team. Although medical students get some experience examining and interviewing patients in the first or second year of medical school, clinical clerkships usually start in the third year of medical school. These students, known as *junior medical students,* spend the year completing required rotations (usually 1 month in duration) in services such as internal medicine, surgery, obstetrics and gynecology, and pediatric services. Their patient workloads are limited to a small number of patients and they are closely supervised by medical school faculty and more experienced team members. Senior medical students, also known as *externs,* are in the last year of medical school. Depending on the medical school curriculum, senior medical students may spend all or part of the last year of medical school in a variety of selective or elective rotations. Externs have more patient care responsibilities than do junior medical students but less than interns or other residents.

The medical team, depending on institution-specific policies, may include a variety of other health care professionals. Some pharmacists provide patient care services to specific patient populations (e.g., critically ill, adult general medicine, pediatrics) and are considered integral members of the medical team. Pharmacy residents, fellows, and students often are assigned to specific internal medicine teams for part of their experiential training. Nurse practitioners may provide patient care services to specific patient populations and attend rounds with the medical team. More commonly, nurse specialists may join the medical team as the team discusses specific patients and patient-specific issues. Some nursing students may be assigned to medical teams as part of their experiential training. Other health care professionals who may be part of the team or join the medical team for rounds on specific patients include social workers, dietitians, medical ethicists, occupational therapists, physical therapists, and respiratory therapists.

The Inpatient Environment

Patients admitted to the hospital are assigned beds on specific floors, wards, or wings (e.g., general medicine, cardiology, orthopedics) according to their specific medical problems. The admitting physician evaluates the patient and orders laboratory and diagnostic tests and medications. The physician may consult with specialty physicians and other health care professionals, including pharmacists. In a teaching hospital, medical residents, interns, and medical students also may evaluate the patient, and the physician of record (the resident or intern) generates patient orders and consults with a variety of physicians and other health care professionals regarding patient care.

The medical record, also known as the *chart,* is a legal document that includes sections for hospital-specific admission and insurance information, initial history and physical examination, daily progress notes made by health care professionals who interact with the patient, consultations, nursing notes, laboratory results, and radiology and surgery reports (Figure 1-2). Most charts include sections for medication orders and other types of orders (e.g., laboratory, dietary, diagnostic procedures); some hospitals maintain a separate ordering system (Table 1-1). All or part of this information may be sorted electronically and be accessible by controlled computer access. When a patient is discharged, the medical record is stored in the medical records department and is retrievable by referencing the patient's hospital admission number.

Many institutions use a recording method known as a *problem-oriented medical record,* or *POMR.* The POMR is structured around a prioritized patient problem list. Physician progress notes and discharge summaries address each patient problem as listed on the patient problem list.

Every page of the medical record and all paperwork that goes to other areas of the hospital (such as medication orders sent to the pharmacy) are stamped with a patient identification number. In most hospitals a plastic card that includes the patient's name, race, address, physician, birth date, date of admission, and hospital admission number is created at admission. A ward secretary (also known as a *ward clerk*) coordinates the processing of paperwork on a hospital unit or part of a hospital unit. Some large units have two or more ward secretaries.

Nursing services are organized to provide 24-hour nursing coverage for all patients. The number of patients assigned to each nurse depends on the severity of illness or disability of the patient and may range from one nurse for one patient in intensive care units to 10 or more patients per nurse on other units. Each floor, unit, or ward has a head nurse with administrative responsibility for nursing services. Some hospitals assign each patient to a primary nurse practitioner who determines the nursing care plan for the patient and coordinates patient care.

Medical team rounds usually occur in the morning. Work rounds, which are led by the resident, usually occur early in the morning. During work rounds the patient's progress is briefly reviewed by the resident, intern, or medical student responsible for the patient; each patient is visited by the medical team. Work rounds allow all members of the team to catch up on the status of each patient and plan for the day's tests, consultations, and other patient care activities.

Attending rounds, which are led by the attending physician, generally occur after work rounds in conference rooms and other areas, rather than at the patient's bedside. Newly admitted patients are presented to the attending physician, who

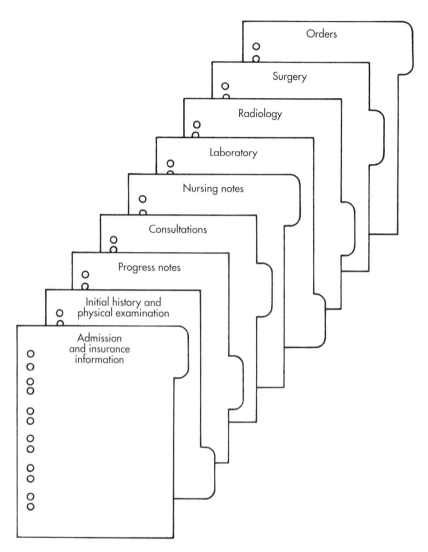

FIGURE 1-2 *Components of the Medical Record.* The medical record contains sections for many types of patient-specific information.

leads the discussion of the differential diagnosis and decision-making processes. Other patients may be discussed in detail, depending on the situation; follow-up information is provided on previously admitted patients. Although some teaching takes place during work rounds, most in-depth teaching discussions take place during attending rounds.

Team members spend the rest of the day independently evaluating patients, assessing laboratory and diagnostic test results, documenting patient findings, consulting with other health care providers, and planning for the care of their patients. The team may gather for radiology rounds, during which radiographs for patients of team members are reviewed. At the end of the day the team gathers for sign-out

Table 1-1	*Medical Record Content*
Section	**Type of information**
Admitting data	Name, address, date of birth, insurance, next of kin
Consent forms	Consent for surgery, procedures, research studies
Physician orders	Medication, dietary, and laboratory orders
Flow sheets and graphic charts	24-hour charts of blood pressure, heart rate, respiratory rate, temperature, and fluid intake and output
Progress notes	Daily physician notes, nursing shift notes, consultant notes
Laboratory data	Blood chemistries, arterial blood gases, cultures and sensitivities, histopathology reports
Diagnostic procedures	Radiology and other diagnostic procedures reports
Consults	Consultant assessments and recommendations
Operating room reports	Preoperative checklist, anesthesia record, graphic records of vital signs, description of events during surgery
Admission history and physical exam	Initial history and physical examination
Medication administration record	Date, time, dose of medications administered; names and initial of nurses who administered medications; lists of all ordered medications
Miscellaneous	Emergency department record

rounds, during which the physician responsible for providing medical coverage in the evening and overnight is briefed about each patient on the service.

The Outpatient Environment

Patients are seen by health care professionals in private offices and clinics by appointment. Some clinics provide "first come, first served" walk-in services; most require appointments. The health care professional–patient interaction is generally short (10 to 15 minutes), except for initial patient evaluations and more complex patient problems and procedures. Patients are referred to affiliated or freestanding laboratory sites for laboratory and diagnostic procedures such as laboratory work, radiographs, and scans; the results are sent to the referring health care provider. Outpatient charts are maintained by the health care provider in a more abbreviated format than that used for inpatients.

THE HEALTH CARE DELIVERY SYSTEM

The health care delivery system in the United States has evolved over the past several decades from a system that held individuals financially responsible for all aspects of their health care to the current system, which advocates society providing equal access and financial support for all components of health care, including access to sophisticated and technologically advanced health care, for all individuals. Many Americans believe that access to medical care is a national right. However, the financial burden of this philosophy has stimulated considerable debate on the best way to use limited health care resources.

Table 1-2	*Public Health Policy Development*
DATE	**ISSUE**
1930s-1940s	Limited support for special patient populations
1940s-1950s	Support for research, facilities, and training
1960s	Broadened health care coverage
1970s	Infrastructure support
1980s-1990s	Cost, quality, and outcomes

From Kissick WL: The evolution of American health policy, *Trans Stud Coll Phys Phila* 11:187-200, 1989.

The health care system is a complex system influenced and controlled by a variety of private and federal factors. Some early attempts at public support of needy individuals date back to the early 1700s in colonial America; however, the prevailing attitude of the time was that individuals, not society, should pay for health care. Health care professionals and institutions were free to charge "customary, prevailing, and reasonable" fees for services; patients paid for private insurance or whatever they could afford if not covered by insurance. The health care system thus evolved to meet the needs of those who could afford to purchase the services. Unfortunately, this type of health care system excluded portions of society and the federal government has had to gradually assume financial and regulatory control of larger portions of the system.[3] Public health policy evolved from a focus on limited support for special patient populations in the 1930s and 1940s to interest in cost, quality, and outcomes in the 1990s (Table 1-2).

Many health care issues remain unresolved. The most pressing of these is the way to decrease the cost of the current health care system while maintaining high quality. Inequities in the health care system are significant; more than one fourth of the population is inadequately insured or completely without health insurance.[4,5] The number of unoccupied hospital beds is large, increasing the competition for traditional and new hospital services (e.g., wellness clinics, fitness centers). An oversupply of physicians is available, but problems with distribution leave many areas of the United States with limited access to health care. The cost of medical malpractice to both the physician and the health care system is high. Defensive medicine accounts for an estimated 15% of the total U.S. expenditures for physician services.[6] Finally, the roles of pharmacists, nurses, and PAs are still evolving, and many questions regarding authority and responsibility for patient care remain unanswered.

SELF-ASSESSMENT QUESTIONS

1 Which of the following is NOT an outcome included in the definition of pharmaceutical care?
   a. Cure of disease
   b. Elimination or reduction of symptoms
   c. Arresting or slowing of disease processes
   d. Prevention of disease or symptoms
   e. Reducing health care costs

2 Skills required for patient-centered pharmacy practice include which of the following?
a. Therapeutic planning and monitoring skills
b. Physical assessment skills
c. Communication skills
d. All of the above
e. None of the above

3 To be eligible for board certification, pharmacists need which of the following?
a. A Doctor of Pharmacy degree
b. Advanced education and training or equivalent experience
c. A postgraduate residency
d. At least 5 years of work experience
e. Three letters of recommendation

4 Board certification for pharmacists is NOT available in which one of the following areas?
a. Pharmacokinetics
b. Pharmacotherapy
c. Nutrition
d. Nuclear pharmacy
e. Psychiatric pharmacy practice

5 Pharmacy fellowship programs prepare pharmacists to become which of the following?
a. Educators
b. Practitioners
c. Business leaders
d. Researchers
e. Administrators

6 Outpatient health care settings include all of the following EXCEPT:
a. Clinics
b. Day surgery units
c. Rehabilitation centers
d. Emergency rooms
e. Private offices

7 Veterans Administration hospitals are which of the following?
a. Public hospitals
b. Private hospitals
c. Federal hospitals
d. City hospitals
e. State hospitals

8 Which of the following team members prioritizes and coordinates the work of the medical team?
a. Attending physician
b. Second- or third-year resident
c. Fellow
d. Senior medical student
e. Junior medical student

9 In teaching hospitals, most in-depth teaching discussions take place during which of the following activities?

a. Sign-out rounds

b. Work rounds

c. Radiology rounds

d. Attending rounds

e. Shift change

10 Unresolved health care issues include which of the following?

a. The way to decrease the cost of quality health care

b. The imbalance between supply and distribution of physician services

c. The role of clinical pharmacists, nurse practitioners, and PAs

d. All of the above

e. None of the above

REFERENCES

1. Hepler CD, Strand LM: Opportunities and responsibilities in pharmaceutical care, *Am J Hosp Pharm* 47:533-543, 1990.

2. Definitions of pharmacy residencies and fellowships, *Am J Hosp Pharm* 44:1142-1144, 1987.

3. Kissick WL: The evolution of American health policy, *Trans Stud Coll Phys Phila* 11:187-200, 1989.

4. Orford RR: Reflections on the Canadian and American health care systems, *Mayo Clin Proc* 66:203-206, 1991.

5. Davies NE, Felder LH: Applying brakes to the runaway American health care system, *JAMA* 263:73-76, 1990.

6. Reynolds RA, Rizzo JA, Gonzalez ML: The cost of medical professional liability, *JAMA* 257:2776-2781, 1987.

CHAPTER 2

Communication Skills for the Pharmacist

LEARNING OBJECTIVES

1 Describe the way to foster two-way communication with patients and other health care professionals.
2 Identify common barriers to verbal communication and describe ways to overcome each barrier.
3 List at least six guidelines for writing medical record notes.
4 State the ways to convey respect for patients.
5 Identify patient situations that may affect patient-pharmacist communication and suggest ways to deal with each situation.
6 State ways to communicate effectively with physicians, nurses, and other pharmacists.
7 Identify skills necessary for effective teaching, platform and poster presentations, and media interviews.

THE ability to communicate effectively and clearly with patients, family members, physicians, nurses, pharmacists, and other health care professionals is an important skill. Some pharmacists are skilled communicators who are comfortable with all types of patients and health care providers; other pharmacists find communication with health care providers in perceived or actual positions of authority and with patients from various socioeconomic backgrounds extremely difficult. Pharmacists with excellent communication skills and average clinical knowledge are more likely to be successful than pharmacists with poor communication skills and excellent knowledge. In fact, the inability to communicate effectively may lead to harm for patients. For example, poor communication between the pharmacist and patient may lead to an incomplete or inaccurate patient medication history or assessment of patient response to therapy, resulting in inappropriate and inaccurate therapeutic decisions. Poor communication between the patient and pharmacist may contribute to patient confusion, disinterest, and noncompliance and may add to a patient's frustration with the health care system. Impaired communication between pharmacists and physicians, pharmacists and nurses, and pharmacists and pharmacists also may harm patients if important information is not exchanged in an appropriate and timely manner.

VERBAL COMMUNICATION SKILLS

Essential communication skills needed for all verbal interactions, including those between pharmacists and patients and pharmacists and other health care professionals, include the ability to listen, understand, and respond to other people's statements (active listening) and the ability to interpret the nonverbal ways in which the other person communicates and respond in a way that encourages continued interaction (evaluation). Environmental barriers to verbal communication should be minimized as much as possible.

Active Listening

Active listening is an important part of communication. Pharmacists need to be able to make other people feel as if they have their full attention. Pharmacists need to focus on other people and the ways they communicate. Interruptions (e.g., telephone calls, beepers) should be minimized or prevented. Pharmacists, who typically juggle multiple tasks and repeated interruptions, must set these distractions aside and really focus on the other person; an open, relaxed, and unhurried attitude should be conveyed.

The pharmacist also needs to be aware of the ways in which patients and health care professionals convey information (Figure 2-1). The tone and modulation of the voice and the number and placement of pauses provide insight into the person's feelings and may reflect on the reliability of the information. Patients who respond with a low level of energy, flat affect, and monotone voice may be depressed. Patients who respond to questions tentatively and hesitantly may not be providing reliable information. Pauses during responses may indicate that the person needs time to recall the information or find the right words. Pauses also may indicate that the person may be censoring the response or preparing to lie.

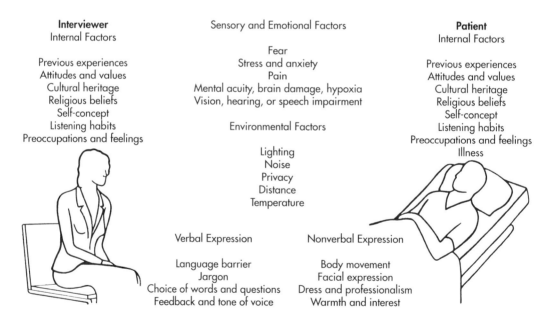

Interviewer
Internal Factors

Previous experiences
Attitudes and values
Cultural heritage
Religious beliefs
Self-concept
Listening habits
Preoccupations and feelings

Sensory and Emotional Factors

Fear
Stress and anxiety
Pain
Mental acuity, brain damage, hypoxia
Vision, hearing, or speech impairment

Environmental Factors

Lighting
Noise
Privacy
Distance
Temperature

Patient
Internal Factors

Previous experiences
Attitudes and values
Cultural heritage
Religious beliefs
Self-concept
Listening habits
Preoccupations and feelings
Illness

Verbal Expression

Language barrier
Jargon
Choice of words and questions
Feedback and tone of voice

Nonverbal Expression

Body movement
Facial expression
Dress and professionalism
Warmth and interest

FIGURE 2-1 *Factors Influencing Communication.* Communication is affected by the integration of patient and pharmacist internal factors; sensory, emotional, and environmental factors; and verbal and nonverbal expression. (From Wilkins RL, Sheldon RL, Krider SJ: *Clinical assessment in respiratory care,* ed 2, St Louis, 1990, Mosby.)

Observation and Assessment

Observation and assessment of the way the other person communicates are important in maintaining the conversation. Body language and gestures can provide important clues for the pharmacist as well as the patient or health care provider. The pharmacist can convey interest and attentiveness by sitting or standing at eye level and maintaining eye contact and body posture. Sitting or standing at eye level or lower projects a nonthreatening, equalizing position that facilitates open communication. The pharmacist should be physically close enough to the patient or health care provider for clear and comprehensible communication but should avoid intruding on the other person's personal space. Invasion of personal space may cause discomfort and be perceived as physically threatening; in either case, communication is compromised.

Pharmacists need to be aware of the nonverbal messages conveyed by patients and health care professionals and change tactics to reengage the other party if the speaker's body language indicates closure to communication. Certain gestures and postures provide information regarding the other person's feelings, although they may not always be accurate (Table 2-1).

Barriers to Verbal Communication

Physical Barriers. Communication across or through physical barriers is extremely difficult. Common physical barriers in ambulatory pharmacy settings include the large countertops and display areas behind which many pharmacists work, windows with security bars and protective glass, and drive-through windows that isolate the pharmacist from the patient. Another common physical barrier to communication in many community pharmacies is the elevated pharmacy area. This elevation accentuates the pharmacist's position of authority and places the patient in an inferior and less comfortable position. Institutionally based pharmacists have fewer physical barriers to contend with than do most community pharmacists, but they have the additional problem of communicating with patients who are in bed. Patients in bed are easily intimidated by people standing over them; interviews may be strained or limited depending on the patient's level of discomfort. The pharmacist can deal with physical barriers by recognizing them and then changing position to allow communication to take place face to face and at eye level or lower.

Lack of Privacy. Lack of privacy is another common barrier to effective communication. Although pharmacists often identify lack of privacy as an issue when

Table 2-1 *Body Language*	
GESTURE OR POSTURE	**IMPLICATION**
Steepling of the hands	Confidence
Raising the hand	Desire to interrupt
Shifting body position	Desire to interrupt
Crossed arms	Shutting out the other person
Leaning toward the speaker	Receptiveness
Raising the hands and then letting them fall limply	Hopelessness
Frequent throat clearing	Disagreement

communicating with patients, it also is an important issue in communication with members of the health care team and other health care professionals; the same approaches for ensuring privacy for patients also apply to other health care professionals. Conversations regarding specific patient information and general health care issues, discussions, and debate must not take place in public areas such as hallways, elevators, and cafeterias.

Patient consultations should occur in privacy. Most community pharmacies do not have counseling areas that are physically separated from the rest of the pharmacy. Most hospitalized patients have at least one roommate; some patients may be in ward settings with three or more patients sharing the same large room. This lack of privacy makes the voicing of personal concerns and the provision of accurate and complete information difficult for many patients. Given a choice, patients tend to withhold potentially embarrassing personal information and avoid asking potentially embarrassing or "stupid" questions if another person might overhear the conversation.

Pharmacists should make every effort to provide as much privacy as possible. Privacy is ensured through the use of a physically separate counseling office. If physically separate space is not available, the pharmacist should converse in a space that is as separate and private as possible. Community pharmacists can maintain a sense of privacy by conversing with patients in a corner of the pharmacy away from the cash register. Pharmacists can maintain a sense of privacy for hospitalized patients by closing the door to the room and pulling the curtain around the bed. If the hospitalized patient can walk, the pharmacist can use nearby conference rooms and vacant waiting areas for private discussions.

The Telephone. Pharmacists must be able to communicate effectively by telephone with all kinds of people, including patients, physicians, nurses, pharmacists, other health care professionals, and relatives of patients. They should project a professional image when communicating by telephone and enhance communication by speaking clearly and really listening to the other person. Pharmacists should provide well-organized information and state facts clearly and calmly.

When initiating telephone conversations, pharmacists should identify themselves by name and explain the purpose of the call. The pharmacist may have to give this information to the person answering the telephone (e.g., receptionist, spouse) and then repeat it when the person being called answers. For example, when calling a physician's office, the pharmacist should say "Hello. This is Joan Arnold. I'm the pharmacist working with Mrs. Johnson. I have a question about Mrs. Johnson's theophylline regimen. May I please speak with Dr. Rivers?"

When answering telephone calls, pharmacists should identify themselves and make sure that they know the identity (name and position) of the caller. They should make every effort to deal with the call and avoid putting the other person on hold. If they are too busy to speak with callers at the moment, pharmacists should tell them that they are too busy to talk with them immediately and arrange to call them back at a mutually convenient time; however, most telephone calls are directly related to patient care and should be dealt with as the calls are received. Interruptive telephone calls should be dealt with in as an unhurried and a professional manner as possible.

Pharmacists sometimes receive telephone calls from angry and upset patients, nurses, physicians, and other health care professionals. The best way to deal with these types of calls is to stay calm, listen to what the person has to say, clarify the issue, and then handle the problem as calmly and coolly as possible. Nothing is accomplished if both parties let their emotions rule the interaction.

WRITTEN COMMUNICATION SKILLS |

Written communication of information is an important skill for all pharmacists. Pharmacists must be able to document patient information in the patient medical record accurately and effectively (charting) and correspond with patients and other health care professionals. Many pharmacists routinely provide written responses to specific drug information questions; this skill is discussed in Chapter 9.

The patient medical record is the primary written communication tool for health care professionals. In the inpatient setting, daily notes are written by all health care professionals involved in patient care. In outpatient settings, health care professionals write notes after each patient interaction. Writing in the patient medical record, or charting, is a privilege that is granted by an institution or organization to specific health care professionals. Many institutions and organizations grant pharmacists charting privileges, although this practice is far from universally accepted.

The medical record is ordinarily used not only to document and communicate information about the patient's progress but also to document the need for remuneration and determine (usually retrospectively) the quality and appropriateness of patient care. Therefore health care professionals must adhere to legal, ethical, and professional standards when documenting patient information (Box 2-1). Contributors to the chart should write in black ink in case the patient record needs to be photocopied (e.g., if it is subpoenaed for a legal hearing); black ink photocopies more clearly and completely than other colors, reducing the risk of the documented information being misread. Clear and legible handwriting and the documentation of factual, nonjudgmental information also are important. For example, the pharmacist may learn during a patient medication history interview that the patient drinks a fifth of whiskey and a six-pack of beer daily. In this situation the pharmacist should document the facts but not label the patient an alcoholic.

Every note in the patient medical record should contain a descriptive heading (e.g., clinical pharmacy, pharmacokinetics, nutrition, attending, cardiology), date and time the note was written, patient-specific information, and the signature of the health care professional. The heading identifies the type of information found

---

Box 2-1 *Guidelines for Writing Medical Record Notes*

1. Use black ink.
2. Write clearly and legibly.
3. Label notes with specific descriptive headings.
4. Provide the date and time on the notes.
5. Document the facts and avoid making unsubstantiated judgments.
6. Organize the information using the SOAP or freestyle format.
7. Sign the note with your name and title.

in the note. This allows other health care professionals to scan the chart quickly for specific types of information. The date and time are important details that allow the information to be interpreted in the context of knowledge concerning the patient at the time the note was written. For example, a pharmacist may assess a patient and make drug and dosing recommendations before all laboratory results are available. Without the date and time, the rest of the health care team may not be able to determine whether the recommendation was made with knowledge of the most recently available laboratory data. The content of the note may be organized using the subjective objective assessment plan (SOAP) or freestyle format (which has no formally accepted organizational structure). The pharmacist should sign the note with signature and title. Notes written by students and other nonlicensed trainees must be co-signed by the preceptor.

INTEGRATION

Communicating with Patients

Effective communication between pharmacists and patients or guardians or family members is extremely important to pharmaceutical care. Ineffective communication may lead to confusion and misunderstanding and may contribute to inappropriate decisions regarding drug therapy.

Patient Titles. Pharmacists should ask patients by which name they wish to be addressed. Unfortunately, health care professionals commonly address patients by their first names, even when meeting patients for the first time.[1] Many patients take offense at being addressed by their first names, especially if they are much older than the health care professional or the health care professional expects to be addressed by title by patients. Addressing the patient by the first name but expecting to be addressed by title puts the patient in an unequal and inferior position and is a throwback to the days of paternalistic health care attitudes. Although some patients who are offended by being addressed by their first names may express their anger or subtly correct the title, other patients may not express their anger but may be unwilling to engage in productive conversation.

Common courtesy dictates that the patient be addressed by title (e.g., Mr., Mrs., Ms., Rev., Dr.). However, the correct title must be used. For example, do not assume that all adult women are married and automatically address every woman as "Mrs." Conversely, do not assume that all adult women, married or single, want to be addressed as "Ms."

The best way to avoid confusion is to ask patients which way they prefer to be addressed. Saying "Hello. My name is Dr. Smith. Do you wish to be called Elizabeth or do you prefer to be called Ms. or Mrs. Sandborne?" requires very little effort. This approach conveys a sense of respect for the patient, lets the patient express a preference, and indicates to the patient the way to address the pharmacist. The one exception to this approach is in addressing the disoriented, confused, or sedated patient; these patients usually respond better to their first names than to their titles.

Respect for the Patient. The pharmacist must display a genuine respect for the patient. To do this, the pharmacist must respond to the patient as a person. However, the pharmacist has to be careful to maintain a professional relationship and avoid exchanging personal information and confidences with the patient, remembering that "An interview is a conversation with a purpose rather than a conversation with a potential friend."[2]

Respect for the patient is conveyed by acknowledging, without judgment, patient-specific attributes that may be different from the pharmacist's value system or even offensive to the pharmacist. For example, attributes such as smoking, excessive drinking, use of illicit drugs, a history of self-destructive behavior, deficient hygiene, and gross obesity may be offensive and difficult to deal with nonjudgmentally. Other patient-specific traits such as beliefs in folk physiology, nontraditional medicine, and unorthodox medical treatments also must be acknowledged without judgment. Pharmacists also must be able to acknowledge differences in socioeconomic backgrounds and ethnic origins.

Respect for the patient is conveyed by the attitude of the pharmacist (Box 2-2). The pharmacist should arrange adequate time for patient interaction and minimize interruptions from telephone calls, beepers, and other patients or health care professionals. The pharmacist should make an introduction, obtain permission to interact with the patient, and explain the purpose of the interaction. Pharmacists who use information obtained from the patient for patient management should explain who will see the information and the way in which it will be used. Pharmacy students who interact with patients should truthfully explain their roles as students and explain who will see information obtained during the student-patient interaction and the way in which the information will be used.

Respect for the patient also is conveyed by the environment established by the pharmacist. The pharmacist should make sure the patient is as comfortable as possible and that as much privacy as possible is provided. In outpatient settings, pharmacists should interact with patients in physically separate areas away from patient traffic areas; they should allow for private and confidential conversation. For hospitalized patients, pharmacists should close the door to the room and draw the curtain around the bed to provide a sense of privacy. When possible, physical barriers to communication should be avoided. The pharmacist should take notes but should not let the process of note-taking control the interaction.

Questioning Techniques. The pharmacist, not the patient, should control the patient-pharmacist interaction. This skill improves with experience in interacting with a variety of patients. The pharmacist can control the interaction by controlling the types of questions asked and the time allowed for patient responses. Controlling the interaction does not mean, however, that the pharmacist should fire off a rapid sequence of yes/no questions and abruptly cut off patient responses.

Early in the interview, pharmacists should ask open-ended questions that allow patients to talk freely about their medications and concerns. This technique lets patients know that the pharmacist is interested in their stories and gives the pharmacist feedback regarding patients' knowledge of their medications and abili-

Box 2-2 *Behavioral Checklist*	
Be relaxed, confident, and comfortable.	Be nonjudgmental.
Show interest in the patient.	Be sincere and honest.
Maintain objectivity.	Maintain control of the interview.

From Zakus GE et al: Teaching interviewing for pediatrics, *J Med Ed* 51:323-331, 1976.

ties to recall and communicate this information. During this period the pharmacist should use minimal facilitators such as "yes," "uh huh," and "what else?" and provide nonverbal encouragement by smiling and nodding when appropriate. The pharmacist should give the patient time to answer. Some patients are able to provide well-organized and detailed information without much additional questioning by the pharmacist; however, other patients may have a tendency to ramble and turn the conversation away from the specific topic of discussion. This is especially true for hospitalized patients who have interacted with a variety of other health care professionals. Some patients may not be able to provide any information without specific and targeted questioning.

After the patient has been allowed to present an uninterrupted story, the pharmacist should narrow the questions and ask more directed and structured questions. The pharmacist should discuss one topic at a time and avoid asking leading questions, multiple questions, and yes/no questions when possible. Simple yes/no questions may be useful in screening for specific information, but if they are used excessively, they shut off the patient's flow of information.

The pharmacist should take time frequently during the patient interaction to summarize the information provided by the patient. This lets the patient know the pharmacist understands, allows the pharmacist to verify the information, and ensures that both patient and pharmacist are in agreement. The use of summaries also lets the pharmacist identify and clarify discrepancies.

The pharmacist should close the patient-pharmacist interaction by providing a summary of the information obtained; the patient should make any last clarifications or contributions. Finally, the pharmacist should thank the patient pleasantly and say "good-bye."

Patient Instruction. Pharmacists have a tendency to consider the prescription label the primary communication tool between the pharmacist and patient. However, optimal patient interaction requires more than this one-way communication tool. Several communication objectives for patient instruction have been identified,[4] including identification of the needs of the patient, control of the timing and amount of information given in each interaction, determination of patient-specific objectives, and assessment of patient learning. For example, the pharmacist should not assume that a patient with asthma who is dependent on steroids understands the way to monitor peak expiratory flow rates with the peak flow meter or the treatment to institute if the flow rates decrease. The pharmacist should question the patient to determine the depth of patient knowledge and understanding and then develop a plan for patient education. However, expecting the patient to absorb large amounts of information from any single interaction is unrealistic. Therefore the pharmacist should plan to convey drug-specific information over several sessions and provide the patient with written information to reinforce verbal information.

The pharmacist must assess the needs of the patient in the context of the patient's emotional status, educational background, and intellectual ability when determining patient-specific objectives. Some patients want to know everything about their medications; others do not want to know anything. The pharmacist should balance the patient's desire for information with the need for information. At the end of the interaction the pharmacist should determine the depth of the patient's learning and retention in a nonthreatening manner. This can be accomplished by asking the patient to summarize or repeat the information discussed. Over time and through repeated interactions, the pharmacist can convey a large amount of drug-specific information and help the patient successfully manage the medication regimen.

Medical Jargon. Pharmacists should avoid medical jargon when communicating with patients. Pharmacists often find avoiding the use of jargon difficult, but they must be able to translate commonly used pharmacy and medical terms into the vernacular and use words patients can understand. Results from a study evaluating patient understanding of commonly used pharmacy terms (Table 2-2) indicated that many patients did not understand these terms; many patients interpreted these terms quite differently than they were intended.[5] For example, some patients thought the term *diuretic* meant a medication for diarrhea or concerned the diet or diabetes; some patients thought the term *generic* meant synthetic or not as good or thought the term concerned the elderly.

Even commonly used medical terms may be misinterpreted by the patient. For example, the term *hypertension* may have different meanings for different patients. Some patients think it means hyperactive or nervous. Some cultures in the United States use the term *high blood* to indicate hypertension and *low blood* to indicate anemia. Other terms such as *angina, divided dose, anticoagulant, sublingual, subcutaneous, intravenous,* and *dyspnea* may have no meaning whatsoever for the typical patient.

The best way to avoid miscommunication and confusion is to speak in plain English and use concrete and specific references. If pharmacists misunderstand patients' questions, they should ask them to restate the message so that both parties understand the topic being discussed. However, pharmacists also should be aware that some patients (especially those with chronic disease, frequent contacts with the health care system, or a health care education or background) may have sophisticated pharmacy and medical vocabularies and may be offended by the use of simple terminology.

Special Situations. Pharmacists must be able to communicate with patients who are unable or unwilling to communicate along generally accepted societal norms. Communication may be compromised by the patient's situation and atti-

Table 2-2	*Commonly Misunderstood Terms*
TERM	**MEANING**
Allergic	A response stimulated by an allergen
Antibiotic	A drug that inhibits the growth of microorganisms
Antihistamine	A medication that blocks the action of histamine
Controlled substance	A medication with addicting potential
Cough suppressant	A medication that reduces cough
Decongestant	A medication that reduces congestion
Diuretic	A medication that increases the amount of urine
Generic	The name for a medication, regardless of its manufacturer
Hypertension	High arterial blood pressure
Inflammation	A complex pathologic process that affects blood vessels and tissues
Oral	Relating to the mouth
Over-the-counter (OTC) drugs	Nonprescription medications
Third-party payers	Organizations that pay health care bills

From Shaughnessy AF: Patients' understanding of selected pharmacy terms, *Am Pharm* NS28(10): 38-42, 1988.

tude. For example, many patients are so stressed by acute or chronic illnesses that they do not (or cannot) adhere to common rules of courtesy. Communication with such patients may be extremely difficult. Differences in ethnic, social, and educational backgrounds may make communication between the patient and pharmacist difficult. The pharmacist, not the patient, is responsible for recognizing the special situation and having the skills and flexibility necessary to ensure appropriate and effective communication.

Embarrassing situations. Most patients are embarrassed to discuss issues related to sex, intimate body parts, and bodily functions (Box 2-3).[6] For example, many female community pharmacists have had the experience of watching men loiter in the pharmacy until they can ask a male clerk about condoms. Many patients are so embarrassed by such situations that they deliberately avoid asking for help, choosing to remain uninformed rather than risk asking an embarrassing question (Figure 2-2).

To deal with these embarrassing situations, the pharmacist must be aware of situations that may embarrass patients and be ready to bring up the subject if the patient has difficulty. The pharmacist also must be sensitive to clues that convey the patient's embarrassment and communicate in a respectful, professional manner. All conversation should take place in as private an environment as possible. In some instances the pharmacist may have to guess at the issue bothering the patient and ask if that is the problem.

Clues to a patient's embarrassment include avoidance of eye contact, blushing, stammering, and excessive nervous small talk about unrelated matters (e.g., the weather, sports). The pharmacist should project a professional demeanor and put the patient at ease by discussing the issue in a straightforward, scientifically appropriate manner. Humor, which may temporarily relieve tension, may make the patient more embarrassed and should be avoided. Anatomically correct terms with clear explanations should be used instead of street slang. Patients should be given many opportunities to express themselves.

Mute patients. Patients may be mute as a result of endotracheal intubation, tracheotomy, or damage to the vocal cords or trachea from disease and trauma. The inability to speak can be extremely frustrating for the patient. The situation can be equally frustrating for the pharmacist, who is accustomed to using verbal communication as the primary tool for obtaining patient information and monitoring the response to therapy. Written communication and point-and-spell letter boards can be extremely time-consuming and frustrating methods of communication. However, they may be the only means of communication for the patient. Pharmacists

Box 2-3   *Potentially Embarrassing Situations*

Asking about drug-induced sexual dysfunction
Asking for any of the following:
• Hemorrhoid products
• Enema supplies
• Douche supplies
• Ostomy supplies
• Birth control products

Discussing any of the following
• Drug or substance abuse
• Alcoholism
• Obesity
• Illiteracy
• Constipation
• Incontinence
• Noncompliance

should encourage these types of communication and allow sufficient time for adequate communication. In addition, pharmacists should maintain their ends of conversations and not limit verbal responses just because the patient cannot speak in return.

Elderly patients. Pharmacists must be aware of the special needs of elderly patients.[7,8] The aging process may leave the elderly patient with limited hearing and vision. The hearing loss associated with aging is characterized by loss of ability to distinguish between high-frequency sounds. This loss may make distinguishing between conversational tones and background noises difficult for the patient. Visual changes associated with aging include loss of accommodation, development of cataracts, reduced peripheral vision, and problems in distinguishing among some colors. These changes may make the patient sensitive to harsh, glaring lights and highly reflective surfaces and may hinder the patient in reading prescription labels

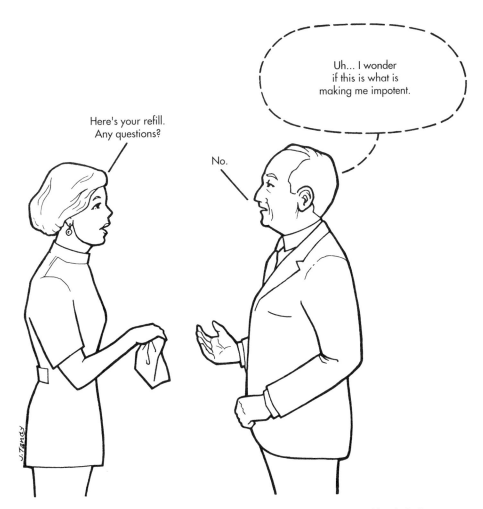

FIGURE 2-2 *Embarrassing Situations.* Some patients are so embarrassed by their situations that they choose to suffer rather than risk public embarrassment.

and other printed material and distinguishing among similarly shaped dosage formulations.

To communicate effectively with elderly patients, the pharmacist must engage in unhurried conversation. The pharmacist should speak slowly, distinctly, and respectfully. Youth-oriented and local slang should be avoided. The pharmacist may need to speak a little louder than usual but should not assume that every elderly person has impaired hearing. The pharmacist should speak directly to the patient and not assume the patient's incompetence or that the person accompanying the patient is the primary caregiver or guardian. The pharmacist should use large-print labels and printed materials and reinforce written information with verbal communication. Touching the patient lightly on the arm or shoulder may reassure the patient and reinforce the content of the conversation.

Pediatric patients. The pharmacist should communicate directly with the pediatric patient as well as with the parent or guardian and should not assume that children have nothing to contribute to their health care. Even young children can begin to understand the purposes of their medications and develop an understanding of the role of the pharmacist; however, the pharmacist must provide information that is appropriate to the age of the child. For example, communication with young children may be as simple as telling them what medications do, whereas in-depth education may be required for the teenager with chronic severe asthma who is using several different medications. Direct communication with preteens and teenagers who have chronic diseases for which they follow chronic medication regimens is especially important. These patients may exert considerable control over their lives, and they need to understand the appropriate use of their medications.

Physically challenged patients. Physically challenged patients often have to deal with multiple barriers to communication.[9] For example, pharmacists, like most other members of society, often have a hard time seeing the patient behind the wheelchair or prosthetic device. Another common barrier is the assumption that physical disabilities are linked with mental disabilities. In addition to these perceptual difficulties, some physical disabilities leave the patient with limited or garbled speech, making understandable expression of information difficult for the patient; other disabilities may impair the patient's vision and hearing.

Pharmacists should communicate with physically challenged patients in exactly the same way as they do with other patients. They should engage patients in unhurried conversation and give them ample time to respond. The pharmacist should speak directly to the patient and not assume the patient's incompetence or that a person accompanying the patient is the patient's caregiver. Moreover, the pharmacist should neither stare nor avoid eye contact and should not physically assist the patient (e.g., by pushing the wheelchair, guiding a blind patient) unless the patient requests assistance.

Mentally retarded patients. The pharmacist must communicate clearly and directly with mentally retarded patients and not assume that these patients are incapable of participating in their health care. The pharmacist should look beyond the disability and deal directly with the patient. However, the pharmacist also must communicate clearly and directly with the patient's caregiver. Many degrees of mental retardation are possible; the pharmacist must be flexible enough to assess the level to which each patient can participate and communicate appropriately for each situation.

Hearing impaired patients. Most pharmacists are greatly impaired in communicating with patients with hearing loss. Pharmacists need to be sensitive to issues in hearing loss and not assume that patients with hearing impairments have diminished intellectual abilities. In addition, pharmacists should not assume that all people with hearing impairments can read lips. Nor should they assume that hearing aids return patients' abilities to hear to normal levels.

Pharmacists may find training sessions on ways to communicate with people with hearing impairments helpful. For example, pharmacists can take courses that teach fundamental sign language skills. Regardless of the level of special skills obtained, pharmacists must make every effort to communicate clearly with patients with hearing impairments. Verbal communication should be slow and distinct and the pharmacist should make every effort to minimize background noise. Pharmacists should face patients who can read lips and avoid turning away from them during the conversation. Written communication may be necessary for two-way communication.

Critically ill patients. The intensive care unit is a highly depersonalizing environment. Patients have little privacy and control over their treatment or surroundings; families and friends may feel overwhelmed and out of control. Patients are frequently surrounded by high-technology equipment and may be sleep deprived; drowsy from pain medication; and uncomfortable from procedures, tests, and surgery. The pharmacist may have difficulty seeing the patient behind the equipment. Nevertheless, the pharmacist should communicate directly with the patient and acknowledge the patient by making eye contact (if possible) and speaking (even if the patient is thought to be comatose) on entering and leaving the patient's room or bedside area. Pharmacists also must communicate directly with the patient's family members, who may be very anxious, frustrated, and overwhelmed by the seriousness of the situation.

Chronically ill patients. Chronically ill patients present unique challenges to communication. As a result of repeated interactions with the health care system or extensive reading about the disease, such patients may be sophisticated health care consumers and may be extremely demanding of information. Some of these patients may know more about the management of their diseases than do many health care professionals; this situation may be threatening for the pharmacist. On the other hand, some chronically ill patients may be completely disillusioned by repeated unsatisfactory interactions with the health care system and may be bitter, cynical, and difficult to engage in conversation.

The pharmacist should be flexible enough to communicate on an appropriate level for each patient. Chronically ill patients deserve the same amount of information and attention as any other patients. Discussing sophisticated therapeutic principles may be a pleasure with pleasant and well-informed patients but a chore with bitter, cynical patients. Chronically ill patients must learn to live with their diseases. This may take many years and may never be fully accomplished.

Terminally ill patients. Terminally ill patients may be sophisticated health care consumers and quite demanding of information; they also may be bitter, cynical, and difficult to engage in conversation. Terminally ill patients may receive complicated drug therapy requiring detailed instruction and monitoring. Some terminally ill patients may require high-dosage narcotics to control their pain.

Pharmacists must treat terminally ill patients with respect and work with them to achieve optimal therapeutic efficacy within the complexities of their illnesses and the health care environment. These patients may need help dealing with complex insurance paperwork and suggestions and guidance on ways to deal with complex medication regimens. Terminally ill patients need close monitoring and reassurance about their medication regimens. For example, some terminally ill patients require large and frequent doses of narcotics. Patients and families may be concerned about addiction; the pharmacist should work with the patient to legitimize the use of the medication.

Hard-to-reach patients. Hard-to-reach patients include those of low socioeconomic status, minorities, and illiterate people.[10] Pharmacists may find communicating with these patients difficult, and the patients may have similar difficulties communicating with pharmacists. Patients of low socioeconomic status may have few resources to deal with health care issues. They also may have little knowledge about health care in general and their own health in particular. They may not have the economic or social resources to participate in preventive health care or manage acute or chronic illness. Pharmacists must be sensitive to these issues.

Pharmacists must look beyond these issues and communicate clearly and directly with each patient as an individual, regardless of the status of the patient. Hard-to-reach patients deserve as much respect, time, and information as do all other patients and should not be glossed over and dismissed because of their social status. Their health needs may be greater than those of other members of society, and pharmacists should be prepared to meet their needs. Pharmacists can help illiterate patients organize complex medication regimens by using different-sized bottles and color-coding the labels. Calendars with dosages of unit-of-use medications stapled to the appropriate date may help illiterate patients adhere to complex medication regimens. Other medication-delivery devices may help patients keep track of their doses. The pharmacist can help financially stressed patients by suggesting alternate, less expensive medications.

Antagonistic patients. Pharmacists may have to deal with antagonistic patients who do not want to be bothered with interviews for medication histories or by monitoring by the pharmacist of their medication therapy. The natural response to these patients is to leave them alone and avoid them if possible. However, these patients deserve as much attention as any other patients and may need more attention from the pharmacist because their behavior alienates them from other health care professionals. The best ways to deal with such patients are to be as professional and direct as possible and limit the length of the interaction to as short a period as possible. These patients may be frightened or simply fed up with the entire health care system; therefore clarification of the purpose of and reasons for the interaction and the ways in which the information obtained from the interaction are used may be helpful. Most patients have a great deal of respect for pharmacists and cooperate if the need for the interaction is clearly defined and they perceive that they are treated with respect.

Noncommunicative and overly communicative patients. Noncommunicative and overly communicative patients present special challenges to pharmacists. Noncommunicative patients never volunteer information or express much interest in what the pharmacist says. These patients answer all questions with unenthusiastic yes/no responses. To facilitate communication, the pharmacist must get the patient to talk about any topic and then ask simple, open-ended questions that will provide at least some of the information being sought during the interaction. For example, patients unwilling to identify the medications they are currently taking may open up and start discussing their medications if asked to describe their satisfaction with past medications. Sometimes no communication method works and the communication remains one way. However, most patients can be drawn out and encouraged to engage in effective two-way communication.

Overly communicative patients digress when asked simple questions. Pharmacists eventually obtain the information being sought but only after investing a lot of time in the interview and learning more details about the patient than is necessary. The best ways to deal with these patients are to take firm control of the conversation from the start and keep redirecting patients who wander off the subject. The patient may have to be allowed to wander a little before the pharmacist gently but politely interrupts the patient to redirect the conversation. For example, a patient may be eager to discuss a pet dog's medical problems. The pharmacist may need to give the patient a few moments to talk about these issues before redirecting the patient back to the focus of the interview.

Communicating with Health Care Professionals

Effective communication between pharmacists and physicians, nurses, and other pharmacists is essential to pharmaceutical care. Poor communication leads not only to frustration and lack of respect among professions, but also may compromise patient care if important information is misunderstood or ineffectively conveyed.

Pharmacist-Physician Communication. Pharmacists and physicians often have trouble communicating with one another. Both professionals are extremely busy; communication may take place when neither party has much spare time to spend in conversation. In addition, pharmacists may have difficulty communicating with physicians because they feel intimidated (Figure 2-3). Pharmacists must be comfortable with their roles on health care teams and confident in their unique knowledge and contributions to patient care.

Pharmacists initiating communication with physicians should be prepared with specific facts and recommendations or have specific questions that cannot be answered by other resources. The conversation should take place in a timely manner and an appropriate location. For example, a physician-patient interaction should not be interrupted for anything other than life-saving questions and information. The interruption of attending teaching rounds with trivial questions and observations better made on a one-to-one basis is inappropriate. So too is engaging a physician in lengthy social small talk when work needs to be accomplished. Confronting the physician with information and questions outside the pharmacist's area of expertise also is inappropriate.

If the physician initiates verbal communication, the pharmacist should be prepared to listen carefully, assess the information or question being relayed, and ask for additional information until the pharmacist has a clear understanding of the physician's concerns. Physician-initiated questions are often vague and general; the pharmacist must clarify terms and issues until the actual question is understood by both parties. For example, a physician may note that a patient's serum digoxin concentration is 0.8 ng/ml. However, this information is useless until the pharmacist finds out the time the blood sample was obtained in relation to the dose of the drug, the time medication was started, the clinical status of the patient, and the goal of therapy for that patient.

Pharmacist-Nurse Communication. Pharmacists and nurses also often have trouble communicating with one another. Both professionals are extremely busy; communication often occurs when neither party has much time to spend conversing. Unfortunately, most pharmacist-nurse communication takes place because of errors in medication distribution systems; much of the tension between the two professions is based on these interactions. Nurses are pressured to obtain and administer needed medication, and pharmacists are frustrated because requests are

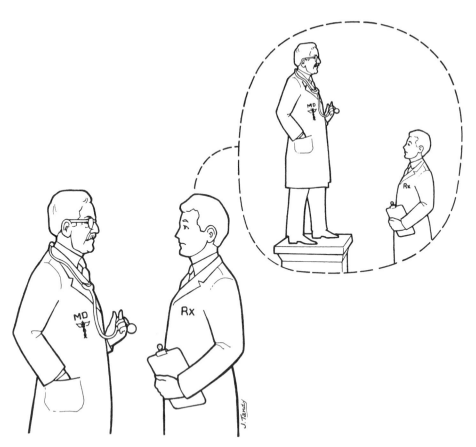

Figure 2-3 *Pharmacist-Physician Communication.* Pharmacists frequently have difficulty communicating with physicians because they feel intimidated.

often presented as emergencies. The pharmacist and the nurse end up in a tug-of-war over work priorities, which can lead to lack of respect and poor communication on the part of both professionals.

An added barrier to effective communication is the use of the telephone as the means of communication. People can easily become quite rude, either intentionally or unintentionally, when dealing with others over the telephone. Feelings may get hurt and reputations lost when tempers are exposed by less than optimal telephone interactions.

Pharmacists and nurses must treat one another with respect; both professionals must realize that they share the same goal (i.e., optimal patient care) and are on the same patient care teams. Communication should be clear, to the point, and timely.

Pharmacist-Pharmacist Communication.   Patient care is sometimes less than optimal because pharmacists fail to communicate patient-specific information to other pharmacists. For example, pharmacists on consultation services such as pharmacokinetics and infectious disease may not have access to the most recent patient information or be privy to team discussions about trends in the patient's progress. Pharmacists on the patient care team do have this information and need to communicate it to all pharmacists providing consultation services to the patient. Consulting pharmacists should be aware that the primary team may have more information than that documented in the patient record; they should not make recommendations in isolation. Patient information can be communicated between pharmacists in informal verbal conversations or may need to be documented in writing.

Many clinical pharmacy services provide services for more than one shift per day 7 days a week. Continuity of service requires that clear communication of patient information, plans for the patient, and other patient issues take place among the pharmacists providing services. A common communication system is the exchange of patient information during sign-out rounds or the discussion of patient-specific issues and the passing on of patient monitoring forms and other types of written documentation between the pharmacists leaving the service and those assuming responsibility for the patient.

One type of pharmacist-to-pharmacist communication that rarely takes place is communication between ambulatory and acute-care pharmacists. The fragmented nature of traditional health care delivery systems at one time made this type of communication nearly impossible; however, unified health care delivery systems may allow for more information to be communicated among pharmacists as patients move between ambulatory and acute-care environments.

ADDITIONAL COMMUNICATION SKILLS

Many pharmacists become involved in a variety of activities requiring additional communication skills. These activities include teaching pharmacy students and other pharmacists, presenting platform and poster presentations at professional meetings, interacting with the news media, and publishing articles in the health care literature.

Teaching

Many pharmacists teach pharmacy students in one-on-one and small group clerkship settings; some pharmacists teach patients, pharmacists, students, and other health care professionals in more formalized classroom and laboratory settings. Although many pharmacists teach, most have had little formal training.

A teacher must be well organized, knowledgeable about the subject being taught, and an excellent communicator. Communication during teaching sessions is enhanced by good organizational skills. The structure of the session and material should be obvious without the use of written handouts. The different sections of the topic should be introduced and summarized periodically. In addition, the teacher should interact with the audience during the teaching session to determine the depth of the participants' understanding and change or redirect the focus of the lecture or discussion to meet the needs of the audience. Direct questioning and assessment of responses are easy ways to determine if the students and participants understand the material; however, these methods are less effective in large classroom settings. Feedback in formal classroom settings comes primarily from nonverbal behavior. Participants who understand and comprehend the material are quiet, focused, and obviously thinking and following along. Participants who are confused or do not understand the material being presented shift uneasily in their seats, converse with those around them, engage in other activities (e.g., reading a newspaper), or fall asleep.

Individual teaching sessions are common clerkship activities. Regardless of the setting (inpatient or outpatient) the student and teacher review individual patient cases and discuss the pathophysiology and therapeutic management of the case. Many students are intimidated by the highly individualized nature of this type of one-on-one teaching; the preceptor should put the student at ease while controlling the educational aspect of the interactions. Students also may feel intimidated or threatened by a constant barrage of seemingly unrelated questions. An effective communication tool during these types of teaching sessions is the circular questioning technique. This technique involves guiding the student through a series of related, basic questions that eventually lead the student to discover the correct answer to a previously asked question. The teacher then asks a series of increasingly difficult questions, allowing the student to reinforce the material already learned and apply and learn new information. Frequent verbal summaries and constructive feedback are essential teaching tools.

Platform and Poster Presentations

Platform Presentations. Many pharmacists present information at local, state, and national professional meetings. However, most pharmacists receive little if any instruction for or experience with these types of presentations. Platform presentations may occur at local, state, and national pharmacy association meetings or may be part of institutional programs. The audience may range from less than a dozen people to several hundred and include pharmacists and other health care professionals. Many people find speaking in public stressful, which in turn may decrease the effectiveness of the communication. Although the degree of stress felt by the speaker depends on the individual and the specific situation, some degree of stress is perfectly natural. Stress is reduced through experience and thorough preparation; however, many experienced speakers still admit to being nervous before and during presentations. Some speakers find they can reduce stress by acknowledging the anxiety rather than denying their feelings. The nervous energy generated by stress can be directed into enthusiasm for the topic and increased energy during the presentation.

Stress can be reduced by appropriate topic selection and thorough preparation. For example, speaking about a familiar topic is much easier than discussing one that is less well understood. Therefore the speaker should be well informed and prepared. Stress also can be reduced by considering the audience and targeting the level of information to the audience's background. This helps create interest on the part of the audience, which in turn provides positive feedback to the speaker. Another way to

Box 2-4	*35-mm Slide Design*

Use simple font styles.
Limit each slide to one idea, figure, or table.
Use a horizontal rather than a vertical format.
Use no more than 5 or 6 lines per slide.
Use a 2:3 horizontal/vertical ratio for each slide.

Use colors to highlight information, but do not use more than 2 or 3 colors.
Use bright, clear colors; avoid pastels and neon colors.
Use simple tables and graphs.

reduce stress is to become familiar with the operation of all audiovisual equipment before speaking in front of the audience. The stress of answering audience questions can be reduced by anticipating and preparing answers to likely questions.

Communication during platform presentations is enhanced by the use of appropriate audiovisual materials. A good visual image can convey information more vividly and accurately than can lengthy verbal descriptions. For example, a videotape presentation of a patient during a seizure provides the audience with visual images that cannot be obtained from verbal descriptions. The 35-mm slide is one of the most common visual aids used during platform presentations (Box 2-4). Other common visual aids include overhead transparencies (Box 2-5) and audiotapes. Computer projectors are becoming increasingly common; they allow for the integration of multiple audiovisual formats, including computer simulations, audiotapes, and videotapes. Visual images should be designed to enhance rather than replace verbally presented information and should be designed so that all members of the audience can see the information.

Poster Presentations. The poster presentation is a unique communication format in which the information is displayed rather than verbally presented. Although most poster sessions require the author to be available to answer questions and discuss the information presented, the visual message conveyed by the poster is what grabs the attention of passersby and draws them in for closer inspection of the details of the presentation. Posters that attract the most attention have attention-getting titles and a colorful, neat, and professional appearance.

The amount of information presented in the poster should be planned in conjunction with the amount of space available for the presentation. The amount of space allocated for each poster varies from meeting to meeting; requirements and limitations are communicated to the presenter when the poster is accepted for presentation. Components of a poster presentation include the title, authors, abstract, introduction and background information, study design, data, results, and references. The printed material should be readable from several feet away. Brightly colored backgrounds enhance the visual presentation. Visual aids such as tables, graphs, charts, and photographs communicate information more effectively than do multiple pages of text.

Media Interviews

Pharmacists may be called by the media to provide background information regarding therapeutic issues such as the marketing of an important new drug or a widely publicized drug-related problem. Media interviews can be interesting and rewarding experiences that provide a positive and effective form of communication between pharmacists and the public. However, pharmacists must ensure that the information provided is understood and not used out of context. Journalists can be

Box 2-5   *Transparency Design*

Use simple font styles.	Use no more than 5 or 6 words per line.
Use letters large enough to be read from a distance.	Use no more than 5 or 6 lines per transparency.
Limit each transparency to one idea, figure, or table.	

quite aggressive. A media expert noted that "if you don't learn to use the media to your advantage, you will be used by it."[11]

Most initial contact with the media is by telephone. The pharmacist should ascertain the name of the reporter, the organization represented, and the issue to be discussed. Pharmacists should not answer any questions, divulge any information, or provide any opinion without knowing this information. Some members of the less-than-reputable media do not offer this information unless specifically prompted. Members of the legitimate media understand the importance of this information and provide their credentials at the start of the conversation.

The pharmacist must prepare for scheduled media interviews by reviewing the subject to be discussed, anticipating related or tangential issues, and being ready to elaborate on and explain technical terminology and concepts in lay language. The pharmacist may wish to speak with other individuals who have been interviewed by the reporter or read articles published by the journalist to get a feel for the person's style.

After the interview, pharmacists need to ensure that material attributed to them is accurate. No one wants to be misquoted; however, being quoted accurately out of context is just as embarrassing. Two ways of ensuring as much accuracy as possible are to be available for clarification, either by telephone or in person, after the interview and to review all printed material before publication.

Manuscripts

Publication of research results and other clinical observations is a common means of communicating information to health care professionals worldwide. Publishing is an important and challenging activity. Successful publication requires excellent writing skills as well as careful planning and execution of the plan.

One of the most important decisions made by the pharmacist attempting to publish a manuscript is the selection of the most appropriate journal. The selection of a journal that publishes the type of material being submitted is most important. For example, editors of the *Journal of Infectious Diseases* would not be interested in publishing a manuscript about a drug used to treat gastrointestinal bleeding. Other common mistakes include trying to publish material and findings already well documented in the literature, submitting a poorly designed and executed study, submitting a poorly written manuscript, and not following journal-specific guidelines. Well-written manuscripts that meet the needs of the journal's audience will be published.

| SELF-ASSESSMENT QUESTIONS |

1 Active listening consists of which of the following tasks?
   a. Focusing on what the other person says
   b. Assessing the way the other person communicates
   c. Conveying an open, relaxed, and unhurried attitude
   d. All of the above
   e. None of the above

2 To convey interest and attentiveness, the pharmacist should do which of the following?
   a. Avoid eye contact
   b. Stand or sit at eye level or lower

   c. Stand or sit as close to the person as possible
   d. Ignore the other person's body language
   e. Take copious notes during the interview

3 Barriers to verbal communication are minimized in which of the following settings?
   a. The interview takes place through a window with security bars.
   b. The interview takes place in front of three of the patient's hospital room-mates.
   c. The interview is conducted over the telephone.
   d. The patient is interviewed in a private consultation office.
   e. The patient is interviewed through a drive-in window.

4 Which one of the following is not an important consideration when writing medical record notes?
   a. Using black ink
   b. Writing clearly and legibly
   c. Titling the note with a specific heading
   d. Documenting the facts and avoiding unsubstantiated judgments
   e. Beginning the note on an unused page

5 When is addressing a patient by the first name appropriate?
   a. When a patient is disoriented
   b. When meeting a patient for the first time
   c. When trying to placate a patient
   d. When a patient is much older than the pharmacist
   e. When a patient is much younger than the pharmacist

6 What kind of questions should be asked early in a patient interview?
   a. Long, complex questions
   b. Questions that can be answered "yes" or "no"
   c. Open-ended questions
   d. Leading questions
   e. Multiple questions

7 Which of the following may make an embarrassing situation worse?
   a. Being aware of potentially embarrassing situations
   b. Being sensitive to clues that the patient is embarrassed
   c. Using humor to relieve the tension
   d. Discussing the issue in a scientifically appropriate manner
   e. Communicating with the patient in privacy

8 The best way to deal with antagonistic patients is to do which of the following?
   a. Avoid them
   b. Suggest less expensive alternative medications
   c. Talk with their legal guardians
   d. Speak slowly and distinctly
   e. Limit the length of each interaction

9 The best way to deal with physically challenged patients is to do which of the following?
   a. Treat them like any other patients.
   b. Avoid making eye contact.

    c. Stare at them.

    d. Ignore them.

    e. Physically assist them without asking permission.

10 Stress associated with platform presentations can be reduced by doing which of the following?

    a. Targeting the material for the specific audience

    b. Acknowledging the presentation as a stressful situation

    c. Anticipating and preparing for audience questions

    d. All of the above

    e. None of the above

REFERENCES

1. How should patients be addressed? *AORN* 31:1142-1144, 1146, 1148, 1980.
2. Ranelli PL, Svarstadt BL, Boh L: Factors affecting outcomes of medication-history interviewing by pharmacy students, *Am J Hosp Pharm* 46:267-281, 1989.
3. Zakus GE et al: Teaching interviewing for pediatrics, *J Med Ed* 51:325-331, 1976.
4. Ivey M, Tso Y, Stamm K: Communication techniques for patient instruction, *Am J Hosp Pharm* 32:828-831, 1975.
5. Shaughnessy AF: Patients' understanding of selected pharmacy terms, *Am Pharm* NS28(10):38-42, 1988.
6. Oliver CH: Communication awareness: Rx for embarrassing situations, *Am Pharm* NS22(10):21-23, 1982.
7. Galizia VJ, Sause RB: Communicating with the geriatric patient, *Am Pharm* NS22(10):35-36, 1982.
8. Portnoy E: Enhancing communication with elderly patients, *Am Pharm* NS25(8):50-55, 1985.
9. Eigen BN: Improving communication with the physically disabled, *Am Pharm* NS22(10):37-40, 1982.
10. Freimuth VS, Mettger W: Is there a hard-to-reach audience? *Pub Health Rep* 105:232-238, 1990.
11. Experts offer advice on dealing with the media, *Mich Med* 89:19-20, 1990.

C H A P T E R   3

Taking Medication Histories

LEARNING OBJECTIVES

1 State the advantages and disadvantages of interviewing patients before and after review of patient information.
2 Identify relevant information that can be obtained from observing the way a patient is dressed and the patient's environment.
3 List the categories of data to be obtained during a medication history interview.
4 Describe the type of information included in each category of data obtained during a medication history interview.
5 Express a patient's smoking history in terms of pack-years.
6 Differentiate between an allergy and an adverse drug reaction.
7 State the way to assess patient compliance with prescribed or recommended medication regimens.
8 Identify types of questions to avoid when interviewing patients.
9 Identify types of patients who are difficult to interview. Describe the most effective ways to interview these types of patients.
10 Discuss the advantages and disadvantages of documenting the patient medication history using a standardized form, the SOAP format, and the freestyle format.

HISTORICALLY, pharmacists have relied on physicians, nurses, and other health care professionals to obtain and document information regarding medications taken by patients. This reliance may have evolved from the general perceptions that this type of information was relatively unimportant and that other health care professionals had more direct patient care responsibilities.

At the turn of the century, many medications were ineffective and did not cause much harm (or benefit); this situation created the perception that medication histories were relatively unimportant in the clinical interview. Unfortunately, this perception provided little incentive for health care professionals to obtain detailed and accurate medication histories. Non–pharmacist-obtained medication histories are generally sketchy as a result, and they lack important information regarding medication allergies and sensitivities, prescription and nonprescription medication consumption, and reliability in taking scheduled doses.[1,2] Recognition of the increasing availability of potent prescription and nonprescription medications and the increasingly fragmented health care system has renewed interest in the need for pharmacist-acquired and pharmacist-documented medication histories.

Information obtained from the medication history is the foundation for planning optimal medication regimens. These data enable all health care providers to generate hypotheses regarding the patient's understanding of the role of medications in the treatment of disease; the ability of the patient to comply with the medication regimen; the effectiveness of the medications; and the patient's experiences with side effects, allergies, and adverse drug reactions. Information obtained from the medication history enables the clinician to judge the effectiveness and tolerability of past and current medication regimens.

Pharmacists have therapeutic and product-specific backgrounds and experience; they are trusted and respected by patients. Although other health care professionals interview patients regarding their uses of medications, no other health care professional has the pharmacist's depth and scope of knowledge regarding medications. Therefore pharmacists must learn the best ways to obtain and document patient medication histories and communicate this information to the rest of the health care team. Obtaining medication histories is not just a matter of common sense and experience. Although interviewing is a creative process that is somewhat difficult to define, successful interviewing requires excellent patient-oriented process skills (Box 3-1) and communication process skills (Box 3-2); pharmacists must be aware of and avoid common hindering behaviors (Box 3-3).

PREPARATION FOR THE INTERVIEW

Regarding preparation for medication history interviews, two schools of thought dominate. One approach is to review all that is known about the patient's medical condition and medications and then target the interview to these areas as identified by previous interviewers. This approach is commonly used when patients are admitted to acute-care or long-term-care institutions in which patient information is readily available. The advantages of this approach are that the pharmacist has some knowledge of the patient going into the interview and can be prepared to explore and address specific questions; the pharmacist may feel more comfortable having this knowledge before interacting with the patient. The disadvantage of this approach is that important information may be overlooked if the pharmacist becomes too focused or unduly influenced by the information.

The other approach is to interview the patient before learning about the patient's medical condition and medication history. Community-based pharmacists rarely have access to information about patients and must be able to conduct effective interviews without knowing the patient or the patient's history. The advantage of this approach is that the pharmacist is completely unbiased about the pa-

---

Box 3-1	*Patient-Oriented Process Skills*

1. Knock on the door and request permission to enter the room of the institutionalized patient
2. Introduce yourself.
3. Try to achieve privacy.
4. Make sure the patient is comfortable.
5. Communicate at eye level or lower.
6. Remove distractions (loud television and radio, relatives and friends).
7. Clarify the purpose of the interview.
8. Obtain the patient's permission for the interview.
9. Verify the patient's name and correct pronunciation.
10. Address the patient by the appropriate title.
11. Maintain eye contact with the patient.

From Zakus M et al: Teaching interviewing for pediatrics, *J Med Ed* 51:325-331, 1976; Lipkin M, Quill TE, Napodano RJ: The medical interview: a core curriculum for residencies in internal medicine, *Ann Intern Med* 100:277-284, 1984; and Preven DW et al: Interviewing skills of first-year medical students, *J Med Ed* 61:842-844, 1986.

tient and the patient's history, thus allowing the exploration of all aspects of the medication history with equal intensity. The disadvantage of this approach is that it can be an intimidating and time-consuming process for the inexperienced interviewer. If all relevant information is not obtained, however, pharmacists can contact ambulatory patients for additional information or interview institutionalized patients again to elicit answers to follow-up questions.

Box 3-2   *Communication Skills*

1. Provide clear instructions regarding the structure of the interview and expectations for the patient.
2. Use a balance of open-ended and closed-ended questions.
3. Use vocabulary geared to the patient.
4. Use nonbiased questions.
5. Give the patient time to respond.
6. Interrupt or redirect as necessary but do not interrupt when the patient is on track.
7. Listen to the patient; do not cut off the patient.
8. Discuss one topic at a time.
9. Move from general to specific topics.
10. Pursue unclear questions until they are clarified.
11. Ask simple questions.
12. Identify and recognize patient feelings. Verbally acknowledge appropriate or hostile feelings.
13. Give feedback to the patient. Ask "Is this what you mean?"
14. Obtain feedback from the patient.
15. Attend to patient cues (posture, tone of voice, affect).
16. Invite the patient to ask questions.
17. Answer patient questions.
18. Use transitional statements and summarization.
19. Close the interview.

From Zakus M et al: Teaching interviewing for pediatrics, *J Med Ed* 51:325-331, 1976; Lipkin M, Quill TE, Napodano RJ: The medical interview: a core curriculum for residencies in internal medicine, *Ann Intern Med* 100:277-284, 1984; and Preven DW et al: Interviewing skills of first-year medical students, *J Med Ed* 61:842-844, 1986.

Box 3-3   *Hindering Behaviors*

Using technical language and medical jargon
Frequently interrupting the patient
Leading the patient on
Allowing frequent external interruptions (telephone calls, beepers)
Expressing bias and personal prejudices
Maintaining a closed posture
Reading notes and charts during the interview
Projecting a superior or threatening posture

Avoiding eye contact with the patient
Engaging in sarcasm
Making derogatory statements about other health care professionals
Ignoring emotion displayed by the patient
Speaking too quickly or too slowly or mumbling
Asking multiple questions
Asking rapid-fire questions
Perpetuating cultural barriers

From Zakus M et al: Teaching interviewing for pediatrics, *J Med Ed* 51:325-331, 1976; Lipkin M, Quill TE, Napodano RJ: The medical interview: a core curriculum for residencies in internal medicine, *Ann Intern Med* 100:277-284, 1984; and Preven DW et al: Interviewing skills of first-year medical students, *J Med Ed* 61:842-844, 1986.

OBSERVATION OF THE PATIENT
AND THE PATIENT'S ENVIRONMENT

Close observation of the patient and the patient's surroundings can provide important information regarding the patient's state of health, compliance with specific dietary recommendations, economic status, and social support system.[6] Each of these factors provides important information regarding the selection, use, and outcomes of specific drug treatments. For example, drugs used to manage hypertension may appear ineffective if the patient refuses to comply with dietary salt restrictions. Patients may choose to pay the rent rather than buy expensive medications. Patients may need help remembering complex medication regimens or may need someone to help prepare and administer subcutaneous medications.

Observations of the way the patient is dressed may provide information regarding general well-being and socioeconomic class. The type, amount, pattern of wear, degree of tidiness, and general fit of clothing should be noted. The amount, quality, and type of jewelry also provides information concerning the patient's socioeconomic status. Worn, dated clothing may suggest that the patient may have difficulty paying for prescribed therapies. Patterns of wear on shoes and shirtsleeves may suggest physical impairment from stroke or other trauma. Long sleeves and broad-brimmed hats inappropriate to the season may indicate photosensitivity or an attempt to hide track marks or scars from suicide attempts. Shoes with toes and other areas cut out may suggest a history of gout or other joint disease. Clothing that is too large may indicate recent weight loss; too-tight clothing may indicate recent weight gain. The pharmacist should note whether belts are buckled at usual wear spots or if the patient has let the belt out or tightened it up. Loose-fitting house slippers or untied sneakers may indicate recent lower extremity edema. A predominance of snaps, zippers, and Velcro-type fastenings may indicate loss of manual dexterity. A patient with hypothyroidism may dress too warmly; a patient with hyperthyroidism may dress too coolly. An unkempt appearance and sloppy dress may indicate that the patient is too ill to pay attention to the details of dressing. Other clues to the patient's lifestyle and sense of well-being include the use of make-up, hairstyle, earrings in men, hearing aids, and watches with large numbers or Braille faces. The pharmacist should, however, not read too much into these observations but should evaluate these observations in context with the rest of the data obtained during the patient interview.

The surroundings of inpatients in nursing homes and long term care and acute care facilities should be carefully noted. Flowers, plants, get-well cards, and children's drawings indicate that the patient has family and friends who are aware of the patient's illness and provide social support for the patient. The presence of books, newspapers, and magazines indicates that the patient can read and provides clues about the patient's reading ability and outside interests. Reading material, crossword puzzles, and crafts such as knitting also indicate that the patient feels well enough to engage in these activities.

The presence of food in a patient's room has several potential meanings. Gift baskets of food indicate social support but may be a problem for patients on controlled and restricted diets. Leftovers from institutional meals may indicate that the patient is not hungry, has missed a meal while at a test or procedure, or dislikes the institutional food. Also, many drugs suppress the appetite and contribute to anorexia. Food from home also may indicate that the patient dislikes the institutional food or that family and friends are trying to supply special foods and treats to entice a patient to eat. The pharmacist should be careful to look for extra or forbidden food in the rooms of patients with diabetes, heavily salted snack food in the rooms of patients on salt-restricted diets, and soft drinks or water in the rooms of patients who are fluid restricted. For these types of patients, dietary indiscretions may be primary or contributing factors in failure of prescribed therapeutic regimens.

DATA TO BE OBTAINED

Data obtained from the medication history interview include demographic information, dietary information, social habits, current and past prescription and nonprescription medications, allergies, adverse drug reactions, and indications of patient compliance with prescribed or recommended medication regimens (Box 3-4). The data obtained should be as complete and descriptive as possible.

Demographic Information

Demographic information includes the patient's age, height, weight, race and ethnic origin, education, occupation, and lifestyle. Lifestyle information includes the patient's housing situation (e.g., boarding house, private home, apartment, shelter,

---

Box 3-4   *Data to be Obtained from a Medication History Interview*

DEMOGRAPHIC INFORMATION
Age
Height and weight
Race and ethnic origin
Residence
Education
Occupation

DIETARY INFORMATION
Dietary restrictions
Use of dietary supplements
Use of appetite stimulants and suppressants

SOCIAL HABITS
Tobacco use
Alcohol use
Illicit drug use

CURRENT PRESCRIPTION MEDICATIONS
Name and description
Dosage
Dosing schedule (prescribed and actual)
Indications
Date medication started
Outcome of therapy

PAST PRESCRIPTION MEDICATIONS
Name and description
Dosage
Dosing schedule (prescribed and actual)
Indications
Date medication started
Date medication stopped
Reason for stopping the medication
Outcome of therapy

CURRENT NONPRESCRIPTION MEDICATIONS
Name and description
Dosage
Dosing schedule (recommended and actual)
Indications
Date medication started
Outcome of therapy

PAST NONPRESCRIPTION MEDICATIONS
Name and description

Dosage
Dosing schedule (recommended and actual)
Indications
Date medication started
Date medication stopped
Reason for stopping the medication
Outcome of therapy

ALLERGIES
Name and description of causative agent
Dosage
Date of reaction
Description of reaction
Way the reaction was treated

ADVERSE DRUG REACTIONS
Name and description
Dosage
Date of reaction
Description of reaction
Way the reaction was treated

COMPLIANCE

on the street), people living with the patient (e.g., young children, elderly relatives, extended family), and the work schedule of the patient (i.e., day shift, night shift, rotating shift schedules, part time, full time). All of these factors can influence decisions regarding selection of prescription and nonprescription medication, the dosage of the medication, and the therapeutic regimen. For example, patients who work with machinery may choose not to take medications that make them drowsy, sluggish, and shaky. Patients who do not have access to rest rooms for lengthy periods may be reluctant to take diuretic medications. Patients who live in shelters or are homeless may not have access to refrigeration. Patients hesitant to give themselves injections may be unwilling to take these types of medications unless a person is available to help them.

Dietary Information

Dietary information includes the type of diet consumed by the patient and dietary restrictions and supplements. For example, patients with diabetes may be following the American Diabetic Association (ADA) dietary guidelines; other patients may be on recommended or self-imposed low-fat and low-salt diets. Some patients may be following weight-reduction or supplemental diets, and some patients may be on low- or high-fiber diets. This type of dietary information must be known because some drugs may appear ineffective if the patient is noncompliant with recommended dietary restrictions. A common example of this type of problem is the patient with hypertension or heart failure who is treated with antihypertensive medications but is noncompliant with a sodium-restricted diet. Additionally, patients may self-medicate with nonprescription dietary supplements and appetite suppressants that may interact adversely with other prescribed medications and treatment regimens.

Social Habits

Social habits include the use of tobacco, alcohol, and illicit drugs. The pharmacist must document the duration of use, amount of each agent consumed, frequency of use, and reasons for use of each agent without being judgmental. The type, quantity, pattern, and duration of alcohol use should be obtained. To assess tobacco use, the pharmacist should note the age at which the patient first started smoking tobacco and when (if applicable) the patient quit smoking. Because the effects of smoking on drug metabolism may be clinically important for weeks to months after the patient has stopped smoking, simply noting that the patient no longer smokes is inadequate. Acute-care pharmacists should be especially sensitive to these issues; patients often quit smoking just before hospitalization and may consider themselves nonsmokers when asked about their smoking habits.

Tobacco smoking is quantified and expressed in pack-years. For example, 1 pack-year is equivalent to smoking one pack of cigarettes daily for 1 year. The number of packs of cigarettes smoked each day and the number of years of smoking are important components of the pack-year history. A 10 pack-year tobacco history may mean that the patient smoked half a pack per day for 20 years, one pack per day for 10 years, or two packs per day for 5 years. Therefore the pharmacist should document the tobacco history in pack-years and packs per day (e.g., 10 pack-year history, two packs per day for 5 years).

Illicit drug use may be difficult to ascertain, but the pharmacist should make an effort to obtain this information in a professional, nonthreatening, nonjudgmental manner. The pharmacist should not try to guess which patients are more or less likely to use these agents but should probe for this information with every patient. Surprisingly, some patients are more comfortable revealing this type of information to pharmacists than they are to other health care professionals, including physicians. Patients generally do not understand the term *illicit;* the best approach is to ask about the use of so-called "street drugs" and give an example or two such as marijuana, crack cocaine, and heroin. The pharmacist should document the amount of each agent consumed; the frequency, pattern, and duration of use; and reasons for use of each agent.

Current Prescription Medications

The pharmacist should obtain a complete description of current prescription medications from the patient. This information includes the name and dosage of the drug, dosing schedule (prescribed and actual), duration of therapy, reason the patient is taking the medication, and outcome of therapy. Knowledge of current prescription medications allows the pharmacist to evaluate the efficacy and safety of prescribed regimens.

Patients may not be able to remember the names of all drugs. If this is the case the pharmacist should obtain a detailed description of the medication, including the dosage form (e.g., tablet, capsule, liquid, topical); size, shape, and color of the dosage form; and any words, letters, and numbers on the dosage form that the patient can remember. If the patient cannot remember the dosage of the drug, the pharmacist may be able to determine this information from other details provided by the patient. However, the pharmacist should clearly document the patient's description and note that the medication might be a specific product. For example, a patient may note taking a small, oblong, bright pink, scored tablet for hypertension. Although this is likely Lopressor (metoprolol tartrate) 50 mg, the pharmacist should document the patient's description and note that the description is consistent with Lopressor 50 mg.

The pharmacist also must obtain the prescribed dosing schedule (e.g., four times a day, two times a day, once a day) and note the routine times the patient takes each dose. If a discrepancy between the prescribed dosing schedule and the schedule the patient uses is apparent (e.g., the patient is supposed to take the medication four times a day but takes it only two times a day), the pharmacist should note the discrepancy and try to determine the reason the patient has elected the different schedule. Patients sometimes change dosing schedules to fit their work schedules and lifestyles or to conserve medication and save money on chronically administered medications.

Many prescription medications are taken "as needed" (prn); as a result, ascertaining the amount of prescription medication consumed by the patient may be difficult. However, the quantification of the use of prescription medications is important and the pharmacist should not accept imprecise descriptive terms. For example, the term *occasional* may mean anything from one dose of the medication every few months to one or more doses per day. One approach to quantifying the amount of medication actually consumed by the patient is to inquire about how often the patient has to obtain a new supply of the medication. This information provides an indirect assessment of the amount of medication the patient actually takes.

The pharmacist should try to determine the exact time or date the patient started taking the prescription medication and the reason the patient gives for taking the medication. Exact dates are important in determining whether an adverse or allergic reaction is a result of a specific medication and whether the prescribed medications are effectively treating or controlling a specific condition. Some patients may not know the specific reason they are taking their medications because they misunderstand the reason it has been prescribed. The pharmacist must document the reasons the patient gives for taking the medication and should clarify any discrepancies regarding usual uses of medications with the prescriber, not the patient.

Past Prescription Medications

The pharmacist should try to obtain as much information about past prescription medications as possible, including name and description, dosage, prescribed and actual dosing schedule, duration of therapy, reason for taking the medication, and outcome. Knowledge of past prescriptions helps the pharmacist understand the medications used, either successfully or unsuccessfully, to treat current and past medical problems; this knowledge guides recommendations regarding new medication regimens. Patients are unlikely to remember this type of information for medications taken in the past; the pharmacist should not get frustrated or frustrate the patient by repetitive "grilling" about these types of medications.

In addition, the pharmacist should document any other information the patient can provide and the reason the patient stopped taking the medication. Medication regimens may be short and well defined, as they are in antibiotic therapy, or multiple medications may be tried over a prolonged period in an effort to find an effective medication with an acceptable side-effect profile.

Current Nonprescription Medications

The pharmacist should obtain a complete description of current nonprescription medications from the patient. Such information includes the name and dosage of the drug, dosing schedule (recommended and actual), duration of therapy, reason the patient is taking the medication, and outcome of therapy. Knowledge of current nonprescription medications allows the pharmacist to determine whether drug interactions may occur between prescribed and self-administered medications, whether the patient is self-medicating an adverse drug reaction from a prescribed medication or in an attempt to obtain better relief from symptoms than that provided with the prescribed regimen, and whether a nonprescription medication is the cause of a patient's complaint or is exacerbating a concurrent medical condition.

Many nonprescription medications are taken prn; quantification of the exact amount of nonprescription medication consumed by the patient may be difficult. However, quantification of the use of nonprescription medications is important; the pharmacist should not accept imprecise descriptive terms. One approach to quantifying the amount of nonprescription medication actually consumed by the patient is to inquire about how often the patient buys a new supply of the medication. This information provides an indirect assessment of the amount of medication the patient actually takes.

Past Nonprescription Medications

The pharmacist should try to obtain as much information as possible about past nonprescription medication, including name and description, dosage, prescribed and actual dosing schedule, duration of therapy, reason for taking, reason for stopping, and outcome. Knowledge of past nonprescription regimens provides the pharmacist with insight regarding past medical problems or attempts to treat current medical problems.

Medication Allergies

The pharmacist must obtain information about medication allergies. Many health care professionals have difficulty differentiating between a true allergic reaction and an adverse drug reaction. The term *allergy* is used to indicate hypersensitivity to specific substances. Drug-induced allergic reactions include anaphylaxis, contact dermatitis, and serum sickness. After a medication allergy has been documented for a patient, the patient will most likely never again receive the medication or any similar medication. If the reaction was a manageable or acceptable adverse reaction rather than an allergic reaction, the patient may be unnecessarily denied access to potentially useful classes of medications.

The identification of true medication allergies may be difficult. A useful first step is to ask patients whether they are allergic to any medications and then probe for the details of the problem depending on the response of the patient. Patients should be asked whether they have ever experienced rashes or breathing problems after taking any medications. Patients may not correlate a rash with an allergy; therefore the pharmacist must obtain the additional information necessary to judge the likelihood of allergy.

After a medication has been identified as the cause of an allergic reaction, the pharmacist should ask the patient to provide details regarding the time or date of the allergic reaction, any interventions instituted to manage the reaction, and whether the patient has received the medication since first experiencing the allergic reaction. The pharmacist also should ask whether medications in similar drug classes have been taken without the occurrence of a similar reaction.

Patients who have experienced life-threatening allergic reactions to medications should be advised to participate in programs such as the Medic Alert program, which provides patients with necklaces and bracelets engraved with patient-specific allergy information.

Adverse Drug Reactions

Adverse drug reactions are unwanted pharmacologic effects associated with medications. Examples of adverse drug reactions include drowsiness from first-generation antihistamines, constipation from codeine-containing medications, nausea from theophylline, and diarrhea from ampicillin. Some adverse drug reactions may be identified by the patient during the discussion of medication allergies. The pharmacist should ask patients whether they have ever taken a medication they would rather not take again. This question often elicits specific descriptions of adverse reactions experienced by the patient. The pharmacist must determine the name of the medication, the dosage, the reason the patient was taking the medication, the details of the adverse reaction, and the way the patient dealt with the reaction (i.e., discontinued the medication, decreased the dosage of the medication, took another medication to treat the adverse reaction).

Compliance

One of the goals of the medication history interview is to determine whether the patient is compliant with prescribed or recommended medication regimens. Knowledge regarding patient compliance is useful in evaluating the effectiveness of prescribed or recommended medication regimens. Medications may be ineffective if the patient does not comply with the prescribed or recommended regimen. Non-compliance may result in additional diagnostic evaluations, procedures, hospitalizations, and unnecessary combination medication regimens.

Compliance is difficult to determine through direct questioning of the patient. Patients know they should be compliant, and if they are confronted by an authority figure, they most likely will say they are compliant even if they are not. Therefore the pharmacist should evaluate the patient's compliance by gentle probing throughout the interview. Clues about compliance may be obtained by descriptions of the way patients take their prescribed medications. Many patients may be able to describe their routines in detail (e.g., setting out a day's worth of doses in the morning, lining up the bottles in a special location, crossing off dates on a calendar); other patients may not be able to describe any sort of routine. Patients who can convincingly describe their medication routines in detail are more likely to be compliant than patients who can only provide vague and general descriptions of their medications and routines.

Sympathetic confrontation may help the pharmacist obtain information regarding patient compliance. If the pharmacist acknowledges that the dosage regimen is complex and difficult to follow or that taking medication regularly is hard to do, patients are more likely to be truthful when describing their difficulties with complying with the regimens. The pharmacist must remain nonjudgmental when assessing patient compliance; this attitude encourages the patient to trust the pharmacist and tell the truth about adherence to prescribed medication regimens.

THE DIFFICULT INTERVIEW

Obtaining medication history information from patients is sometimes difficult. Some patients are especially difficult to interview. Recalcitrant patients, verbose patients, confused patients, patients whose command of the English language is limited, patients with hearing impairments, patients with aphasia, impatient patients, and patients hospitalized in isolation rooms all may be difficult to interview. Although these types of patients may intimidate even the most experienced interviewer, the pharmacist must try to obtain an accurate medication history.

Many interventions are possible. The best approach for recalcitrant or verbose patients is to exert firm control of the interview and ask directed questions to draw information from the recalcitrant patient and redirect the verbose patient. The confused or aphasic patient may not be able to provide any specific information. In this situation, the pharmacist should try to interview family members and friends of the patient. Interpreters are available for many foreign languages in most institutions; pharmacists should use these resources in addition to interviewing family members and friends of the patient. Communication with patients with hearing impairments may be enhanced by ensuring that the patient's hearing aid (if any) is turned on, speaking more clearly and distinctly, and sharing written information with the patient. The impatient patient should be reminded of the need to obtain an accurate medication history; the pharmacist should make every attempt to obtain the history efficiently and in a reasonable amount of time.

The process for interviewing patients in isolation rooms (e.g., respiratory isolation, enteric isolation, infectious disease isolation) is the same as is the process for interviewing any other hospitalized patient with the exception that the pharmacist must comply with all precautions (e.g., wearing masks, gowns, gloves) posted outside the patient's room. The pharmacist should be aware that these precautions may present barriers to communication and should make every effort to overcome them. However, pharmacists may find these patients especially eager to be interviewed because isolation prevents much of the casual human contact that routinely takes place with institutionalized patients.

QUESTIONING TECHNIQUES

The pharmacist should ask open-ended questions at the start of the interview and then move to more direct and targeted questions as the interview proceeds. For example, a good opening question is to ask the patient to describe the medication taken every day. This technique allows the patient to relate the medication regimen routine and provides the pharmacist with clues regarding which lines of targeted questioning should be pursued later in the interview. An example of a more direct and targeted question is to ask the patient to describe the size, shape, and color of the medication regularly taken. Every patient is different, so the pharmacist must be flexible and guide the patient through the interview.

Pharmacists should avoid asking leading questions, multiple questions, and excessive yes/no questions. Leading questions such as "Does your tuberculosis medication turn your urine red?" may make the patient think the medication is supposed to do this and that something is wrong if the patient answers negatively. The pharmacist should probe for these types of medication-related effects by asking more general questions such as "How are you tolerating your tuberculosis medications?" The pharmacist must avoid the easy trap of getting into a pattern of asking a series of rapid-fire questions without giving the patient time to answer. The patient should have ample time to address each question before being asked another. Getting into a pattern of asking a series of yes/no questions also is very easy, especially toward the end of the interview, when the pharmacist asks specific and targeted questions. Such a series might include questions such as "Do you take anything for headache? Do you take anything for your eyes? Do you take anything for your heart? Do you take anything for your breathing? Do you take anything when you have a cold? Have you ever taken penicillin?" These types of rapid-fire yes/no questions create one-sided conversations and may diminish the flow of information from the patient. Patients should be encouraged to talk about their experiences with medications.

DOCUMENTATION OF THE MEDICATION HISTORY

The details of the medication history must be documented in writing and communicated to the health care team. Many standardized patient profile forms have specific areas for the documentation of this information. Some institutions use standardized medication history forms that are filled out, signed, and placed in the patient medical record (Figure 3-1). These standardized forms are relatively easy to fill out and are easy to scan for specific information. However, standardized forms are inflexible and may not provide adequate space for documentation of patient-specific information. Direct documentation of the medication history in the patient record using either the subjective objective assessment plan (SOAP) format or a freestyle format allows individualization of the documentation of each history.

Medication History

Patient: ___John Smith_____   Date: ___1/31/97   1300___

Pharmacist: ___Jane Doe, PharmD_____

Date of Admission: ___1/31/97_____ Room: ___1221b_____ ID Number: ___8963011___

DOB: ___12-3-35_____ Gender: ___M_____ Height: ___5' 11"_____ Weight: ___185 lbs.____

Current Prescription Medications (generic/trade names, starting date, dose, schedule, indication):
   Disopyramide (Norpace®) 200 mg po q 6 h × 2 wks "for heart," is not working
   Captopril (Capoten®) 25 mg po TID × about 10 yrs for HTN; controls BP
   Warfarin (Coumadin®) 5 mg po qd; started 12-15-96; to "prevent clots"
   Digoxin (Lanoxin®) 0.25 mg po qd; started 12-15-96; to "slow down heart"

Past Prescription Medications (generic/trade names, start/stop dates, dose, schedule, indication):
   Quinidine gluconate (Quinaglute®) 324-648 mg po TID in 12/96 for "rapid heart"; exact dates
      unclear; did not work
   Procainamide (Procan®) 500 mg po q 6 h × 3 days in 12/96 for "rapid heart"; exact dates unclear;
      did not work
   EC ASA (Ecotrin®) 325 mg po daily × about 5 yrs to prevent heart attacks; stopped 12-15-96 when
      warfarin (Coumadin®) started

Current Nonprescription Medications (generic/trade names, starting date, dose, schedule, indication):
   Simethicone (Mylicon®) unknown dose (described as one small white tablet) PRN gas; rare use; buys
      one box every couple of years; has used for "years"; very effective
   Acetaminophen (Tylenol®) 650 mg po PRN HA; rare use; takes 1-2 doses about 6 times per year ×
      "many years"; very effective

Past Nonprescription Medications (generic/trade names, start/stop dates, dose, schedule, indication):
   None

Allergies (generic/trade names, date, description of event, treatment):
   NKDA

Social History (tobacco, alcohol, illicit drugs, occupation, housing):
   Accountant; lives in own home with wife
      + Tobacco (1 ppd × 40 yrs)
      + Alcohol (one six-pack of beer per week × 40 years)
      Denies use of illicit drugs

Dietary Information (restrictions, supplements):
   NAS diet × "years"

Assessment of Patient Compliance:
   Patient knows his medications and seems to be compliant. He is eager to have his atrial
   fibrillation under control and is willing to try any medication.

Plan:
   Continue the digoxin (Lanoxin®), warfarin (Coumadin®), and captopril (Capoten®). Check the most
   recent INR and serum digoxin concentration; adjust as necessary. Proceed with propafenone
   (Rythmol®) as planned. Monitor for increased serum digoxin concentrations when propafenone
   (Rythmol®) added and adjust the digoxin (Lanoxin®) dose as necessary. Consider alternate medications such as low-dose amiodarone (Amrinone®) if propafenone (Rhythmol®) or electrical cardioversion do not convert to NSR.

FIGURE 3-1 *Medication History—Standardized Form.* Standardized forms are easy to fill
out but are inflexible.

In the SOAP format, the medication history information is organized into sections (Figure 3-2). This format produces well-organized information but is somewhat repetitive and tedious. In the freestyle format, medication history information is organized in the structure the pharmacist thinks best for the information (Figure 3-3). The freestyle format is easy to write but may make finding specific details difficult; necessary information is more likely to be left out in this format than it is with other formats.

1/31/97   1300   **Medication History**

S: "Rapid heart."

O: John Smith is a 62 y/o WM (DOB 12-3-35) with HTN × 10 yrs and recent onset atrial fibrillation noted on routine physical exam last month. He failed trials of quinidine (Quinaglute®), disopyramide (Norpace®), and procainamide (Procan®). He is admitted for a trial of propafenone (Rythmol®). Electrical cardioversion is planned if propafenone (Rythmol®) does not work. He is 5' 11" and weighs 185 lbs. He has NKDA and no known adverse drug reactions. He is currently smoking and has a 40-year smoking history (1 ppd × 40 years). He drinks a six-pack of beer per week and has done so for 40 years. He denies illicit drug use. He is an accountant and lives in his home with his wife. He tries to limit his salt intake (no added salt at the table).

      His current prescription medications include disopyramide (Norpace®) 200 mg po every 6 hours × 2 weeks "for heart," captopril (Capoten®) 25 mg po TID for about 10 years for HTN, warfarin (Coumadin®) 5 mg po daily to "prevent clots" (started 12-15-96), and digoxin (Lanoxin®) 0.25 mg po daily to "slow down heart" (started 12-15-96). The Norpace® is not working. The Capoten® is controlling his BP. His past prescription medications include quinidine gluconate (Quinaglute®) 324-648 mg po TID in 12/96 for "rapid heart" (exact dates and doses unclear; did not work), procainamide (Procan®) 500 mg po every 6 hours × 3 days in 12/96 for "rapid heart"; taken after quinidine but exact dates unclear; did not work.

      His current nonprescription medications include simethicone (Mylicon®) unknown dose (one small white tablet) PRN gas (buys one box every couple of years; very effective), acetaminophen (Tylenol®) 650 mg PRN HA (takes 1-2 doses about 6 times per year and has done so for "many years"; very effective). He used to take EC ASA (Ecotrin®) 325 mg po daily. He took EC ASA (Ecotrin®) for about 5 years to prevent heart attacks until it was stopped 12-15-96 when the warfarin (Coumadin®) was started. He has not taken any other nonprescription medications.

A: Patient has an excellent knowledge regarding the medications he has taken. He is eager to have his atrial fibrillation under control and claims to take all medications exactly as prescribed. His blood pressure is adequately controlled with the current regimen.

P: Continue the digoxin (Lanoxin®), warfarin (Coumadin®), and captopril (Capoten®). Check the most recent INR and serum digoxin concentration; adjust as necessary. Proceed with propafenone (Rythmol®) as planned. Monitor for increased serum digoxin concentrations when propafenone (Rythmol®) is added and adjust the digoxin (Lanoxin®) as necessary, If propafenone or electrical cardioversion are ineffective, consider a trial of alternate medications such as low-dose amiodarone (Amrinone®).

                              Jane Doe, PharmD

FIGURE 3-2 *Medication History—SOAP Format.* The SOAP format produces well-organized information but is somewhat repetitive and tedious.

1/31/97   1300   **Medication History**

John Smith is a 62-year-old WM (DOB 12-2-35) with a PMH significant for HTN × 10 years and recent onset atrial fibrillation described as "rapid heart" noted on routine physical exam in 12/96. He was initially started on a trial of quinidine (Quinaglute®) which failed to convert him back to NSR. Disopyramide (Norpace®) and procainamide (Procan®) were tried but also failed to convert him to NSR. He is being admitted for a trial with propafenone (Rythmol®); electrical cardioversion will be tried if propafenone (Rythmol®) fails. 5′ 11″, 185 lbs.

SH: Accountant; lives in own home with wife
+ Tobacco (1 ppd × 40 yrs)
+ Alcohol (One six-pack of beer per week × 40 years)
Denies illicit drugs

Dietary: NAS

Allergies: NKDA

ADRs: None

Current Prescription Medications:
Disopyramide (Norpace®) 200 mg po every 6 hours × 2 weeks "for heart"; is not working
Captopril (Capoten®) 25 mg po TID × about 10 years for HTN; controls BP

Past Prescription Medications:
Quinidine gluconate (Quinaglute®) 324-648 mg TID in 12/96 for "rapid heart"; exact dates unclear; did not work
Procainamide (Procan®) 500 mg po every 6 hours × 3 days in 12/94 for "rapid heart"; taken after Quinaglute® but exact dates unclear; did not work

Current Nonprescription Medications:
Simethicone (Mylicon®) unknown dose (one small white tablet) PRN gas; rare use (buys one box every couple of years); very effective
Acetaminophen (Tylenol®) 650 mg PRN HA; rare use; takes 1-2 doses about 6 times per year × "many years"; very effective

Past Nonprescription Medications:
EC ASA (Ecotrin®) 325 mg po daily × about 5 years to prevent heart attacks; stopped 12/15/96 when warfarin (Coumadin®) started

The patient is a pleasant man and a good historian. He knows his medications well and appears to be very compliant. He is eager to have his atrial fibrilllation under control and is willing to try any medication. My plan for the patient is to continue with his current antihypertensive medication, which is providing good control of his BP. Continue the digoxin (Lanoxin®) and coumadin (Warfarin®) but check the most recent INR and serum digoxin concentration and adjust the doses as necessary. Proceed with propafenone (Rythmol®) as planned. Monitor for increased serum digoxin concentrations with the addition of propafenone (Rythmol®). If propafenone (Rythmol®) or subsequent electrical conversion do not control his atrial fibrillation, consider a trial of alternate medications such as low-dose amiodarone (Amrinone®).

Jane Doe, PharmD

FIGURE 3-3 *Medication History—Freestyle Format.* The freestyle format makes writing specific information easy but finding information difficult.

| **Box 3-5** | *Medication History Checklist* |

☐ The date and time of the interview are noted.

☐ The history is signed (and co-signed if entries were made by a student).

☐ The history is written in black ink.

☐ The history includes an appropriate heading (e.g., Medication History)

☐ All medications are referred to by generic and (if applicable) trade names; a complete description of the dosage form is provided if name not known.

☐ The start date is noted for all medications.

☐ The stop date is noted for all past medications.

☐ The dosage and interval is noted for all medications.

☐ The actual use of each daily medication and social drug is noted ("as needed" and "occasional" are not acceptable descriptions).

EACH OF THE FOLLOWING COMPONENTS IS INCLUDED:

☐ Patient demographics

☐ Current prescription medications

☐ Past prescription medications

☐ Current nonprescription medications

☐ Past nonprescription medications

☐ Indications for each medication

☐ Medication allergies

☐ Adverse drug reactions

☐ Dietary information

☐ Social drug information

☐ Assessment of compliance

Regardless of the format used to document the information, every component of the medication history must be included, details should be complete and precisely documented, generic and trade names (where appropriate) should be documented, and handwriting must be clear and readable. The pharmacist may wish to use a checklist when documenting the history (Box 3-5).

SELF-ASSESSMENT QUESTIONS

1 Which of the following is a disadvantage of reviewing all available information about a patient before interviewing the patient?
   a. The pharmacist feels more comfortable.
   b. The pharmacist is prepared to address specific issues.
   c. The pharmacist may be too focused and overlook important issues.
   d. The pharmacist is completely unbiased about all aspects of the history.
   e. This can be a very intimidating process.

2 During a patient interview the pharmacist observes that the patient's clothing has a predominance of Velcro-type fastenings. This may indicate which of the following?
   a. Photosensitivity
   b. Recent weight loss
   c. Recent weight gain
   d. Loss of manual dexterity
   e. Gout

3 Demographic patient information includes all of the following EXCEPT:
   a. Age
   b. Height
   c. Weight
   d. Ethnic origin
   e. Dietary restrictions

4 A patient states that he has smoked two packs of cigarettes a day for 30 years. What is the patient's pack-year smoking history?
   a. 2 pack-years
   b. 15 pack-years
   c. 30 pack-years
   d. 60 pack-years
   e. 90 pack-years

5 Current prescription information includes all of the following EXCEPT:
   a. The name and description of the drug
   b. The date or time the medication was stopped
   c. The dosage of the drug
   d. The prescribed and actual dosing schedule
   e. The date or time the medication was started

6 What information should be documented regarding a suspected medication allergy?
   a. The date or time the reaction occurred
   b. The interventions performed to manage the reaction
   c. Whether the patient has received similar medications
   d. All of the above
   e. None of the above

7 Which of the following questioning techniques is LEAST likely to result in an accurate assessment of patient compliance?
   a. Direct questioning
   b. Gentle probing
   c. Sympathetic confrontation
   d. Nonjudgmental questioning
   e. Asking the patient to describe the daily routine

8 In general, which of the following types of questions should be avoided when interviewing patients?
   a. Leading questions
   b. Multiple questions
   c. Excessive yes/no questions
   d. All of the above
   e. None of the above

9 Which of the following is the best approach to interviewing verbose patients?
   a. Asking directed questions
   b. Interviewing family members
   c. Using an interpreter
   d. Speaking slowly and loudly
   e. Interviewing friends

10 Which one of the following is a disadvantage of documenting a medication history using the freestyle format?
  a. The format is inflexible.
  b. Scanning the document for specific details is difficult.
  c. Space may not be available for all patient information.
  d. All of the above
  e. None of the above

REFERENCES

1. Wilson RS, Kabat HF: Pharmacist initiated patient drug histories, *Am J Hosp Pharm* 28:49-53, 1971.
2. Covington TR, Pfeiffer FG: The pharmacist-acquired medication history, *Am J Hosp Pharm* 29:692-695, 1972.
3. Zakus M et al: Teaching interviewing for pediatrics, *J Med Ed* 51:325-331, 1976.
4. Lipkin M, Quill TE, Napodano RJ: The medical interview: a core curriculum for residencies in internal medicine, *Ann Intern Med* 100:277-284, 1984.
5. Preven DW et al: Interviewing skills of first-year medical students, *J Med Ed* 61:842-844, 1986.
6. Fitzgerald FT, Tierney LM: The bedside Sherlock Holmes, *West J Med* 137:169-175, 1982.

C H A P T E R   4

Physical Assessment Skills

LEARNING OBJECTIVES

1 List the four fundamental physical assessment techniques and describe the way to perform each of the techniques.
2 Identify the components of the stethoscope, ophthalmoscope, and otoscope and state the way each is used to assess patients.
3 Describe the use of the tuning fork and reflex hammer to assess patients.
4 Describe the way to assess each of the major organ systems.
5 Define common physical assessment terms.
6 Interpret common physical assessment abbreviations.

PHARMACISTS use laboratory data and information obtained from the physical examination and patient interview to assess response to drug and nondrug therapy. Although the need for hands-on proficiency in specific physical assessment skills varies according to the type of patient care setting, all pharmacists should have at least a basic understanding of these skills. At a minimum they should be able to decipher common physical assessment abbreviations (Table 4-1) and interpret and assess specific findings reported by other health care professionals. Pharmacists in some clinical settings (e.g., ambulatory clinics) routinely assess patients using a wide variety of physical assessment skills. Although the practice settings requiring proficiency in a broad range of physical assessment skills are currently relatively few in number, the need for these skills continues to grow as pharmacists assume more direct patient-care responsibilities.

This chapter introduces the pharmacist to the processes, techniques, and components of the physical examination. However, physical examination is a complex process that requires significant effort and experience to master. Pharmacists interested in learning more about the physical examination should refer to one or more of the excellent in-depth physical examination textbooks available in medical libraries and bookstores. Additionally, an increasing number of hands-on continuing education courses are available for pharmacists.

THE PROCESS

The patient's privacy must be respected and patient discomfort and embarrassment minimized. The examination, usually conducted from the patient's right side, follows a generally accepted sequence that minimizes the number of changes in position by the patient and clinician (Box 4-1). The scope of the examination varies depending on the patient's illness and its severity. For example, a thorough and detailed examination of all organ systems must be performed in the evaluation of a severely ill patient with multiple complaints; subsequent examinations may tar-

| **Table 4-1** | *Common Physical Assessment Abbreviations* |

ABBREVIATION	MEANING	ABBREVIATION	MEANING
ABDOMINAL		CVAT	Costovertebral angle tenderness
Abd	Abdomen	DP	Dorsalis pedis
BRBPR	Bright red blood per rectum	FROM	Full range of motion
BS	Bowel sounds	LE	Lower extremity
CM	Costal margin	LLE	Left lower extremity
HJR	Hepatojugular reflux	LUE	Left upper extremity
HSM	Hepatosplenomegaly	PT	Popliteal
LCM	Left costal margin	RLE	Right lower extremity
LLQ	Left lower quadrant	ROM	Range of motion
LUQ	Left upper quadrant	RUE	Right upper extremity
NABS	Normal active bowel sounds	Tr	Trace
NTND	Nontender, nondistended	UE	Upper extremity
RCM	Right costal margin		
RLQ	Right lower quadrant	**GENERAL**	
RUQ	Right upper quadrant	ABW	Actual body weight
		AF	Asian female
CARDIOVASCULAR		AM	Asian male
AI	Aortic insufficiency	$A\&O \times 3$	Awake and oriented to person, place, and time
AR	Aortic regurgitation		
AS	Aortic stenosis	A&P	Auscultation and percussion
5ICSMCL	Fifth intercostal space midclavicular line	A&W	Alive and well
		BF	Black female
CV	Cardiovascular	BM	Black male
JVD	Jugular venous distention	BP	Blood pressure
JVP	Jugular venous pressure	BPM	Beats per minute; breaths per minute
LLSB	Left lower sternal border		
M	Murmur	Bx	Biopsy
MAP	Mean arterial pressure	DBP	Diastolic blood pressure
MR	Mitral regurgitation	HF	Hispanic female
MRG	Murmurs, rubs, gallops	HM	Hispanic male
MS	Mitral stenosis	HR	Heart rate
MVP	Mitral valve prolapse	IBW	Ideal body weight
NSR	Normal sinus rhythm	LBW	Lean body weight
OS	Opening snap	AAF	African-American female
PMI	Point of maximal impulse	AAM	African-American male
RRR	Regular rate and rhythm	NAD	No acute distress; no apparent disease
S_1	First heart sound		
S_2	Second heart sound	PE	Physical examination
S_3	Third heart sound	PPD	Packs per day
S_4	Fourth heart sound	SBP	Systolic blood pressure
SEM	Systolic ejection murmur	T	Temperature
USB	Upper sternal border	$T_{(a)}$	Temperature, axillary
		$T_{(po)}$	Temperature, oral
EXTREMITIES		$T_{(R)}$	Temperature, rectal
AKA	Above-knee amputation	$T_{(T)}$	Temperature, tympanic
BKA	Below-knee amputation	VS	Vital signs
CCE	Cyanosis, clubbing, and edema	VSS	Vital signs stable
CVA	Costovertebral angle		

Continued

Table 4-1 Common Physical Assessment Abbreviations—cont'd

ABBREVIATION	MEANING	ABBREVIATION	MEANING
WDWN	Well developed, well nourished	Bab	Babinski reflex
WF	White female	BC	Bone conduction
WM	White male	BC > AC	Bone conduction greater than air conduction
WNL	Within normal limits	CN	Cranial nerve
Y/O	Years old	CN II-XII	Cranial nerves two through twelve
HEAD, EYES, EARS, NOSE, AND THROAT		DTR	Deep tendon reflexes
C/D	Cup-to-disc ratio	FTN	Finger-to-nose
EOMI	Extraocular muscles intact	HTS	Heel-to-shin
HEENT	Head, eyes, ears, nose, and throat	MS	Mental status
		MSE	Mental status examination
IOP	Intraocular pressure	NM	Neuromuscular
NCAT	Normocephalic, atraumatic	PP	Pinprick
NR	Nonreactive	RAM	Rapid alternating movements
OD	Right eye		
OS	Left eye	**PULMONARY**	
PERRLA	Pupils equal, round, and reactive to light and accommodation	AP	Anteroposterior
		BS	Breath sounds
		CTA	Clear to auscultation
SCM	Sternocleidomastoid	E→A	Egophony
SHEENT	Skin, head, eyes, ears, nose, and throat	LLL	Left lower lobe
		LUL	Left upper lobe
TM	Tympanic membrane	PA	Posteroanterior
		RLL	Right lower lobe
NEUROLOGIC		RML	Right middle lobe
AC	Air conduction	RR	Respiratory rate
AC > BC	Air conduction greater than bone conduction	RUL	Right upper lobe

Box 4-1 The Usual Physical Assessment Sequence

1. Vital signs
2. Appearance and behavior
3. Skin
4. Head
5. Eyes
6. Ears
7. Nose
8. Mouth
9. Neck
10. Breasts
11. Chest and lungs
12. Heart
13. Abdomen
14. Extremities
15. Back and spine
16. Nervous system
17. Mental status
18. Genitalia and rectum

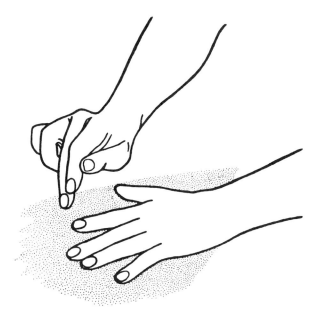

FIGURE 4-1 *Percussion.* Technique for indirect percussion. Only the pleximeter finger contacts the body. (From Wilkins RL, Sheldon RL, Krider SJ, editors: *Clinical assessment in respiratory care,* ed 2, St Louis, 1990, Mosby.)

get specific organ systems with perfunctory assessment (if any) of the other organ systems. The usual neurologic examination is a simple screening examination unless otherwise indicated.

THE TECHNIQUES

The physical examination consists of a detailed patient evaluation using the four fundamental techniques of inspection, percussion, palpation, and auscultation (IPPA). Inspection denotes visual surveillance. For example, the skin is inspected for color and the presence of lesions, visible trauma, and other abnormalities. Percussion is used to determine the density of a specific area or part of the body. A percussion note is created by either tapping the body directly with the distal end of a finger (direct percussion) or by tapping a finger placed on the body (indirect percussion) (Figure 4-1). Only the finger being struck should touch the body. Percussion over normal lung tissue produces a resonant, hollow sounding percussion note; percussion over solid organs (e.g., the liver) produces a dull percussion note. Palpation consists of using the hands to feel body parts that cannot be seen to aid in diagnosis. For example, palpation is used to feel the lower edge of the liver and locate the spleen tip. Auscultation consists of listening either directly with the ear or indirectly with the aid of a device (typically a stethoscope) to sounds that arise spontaneously from the body (e.g., breath sounds, heart sounds, bowel sounds, bruits).

EQUIPMENT

Several pieces of equipment are required for the physical examination (Table 4-2).

The stethoscope, an important auscultatory tool, consists of two ear pieces angled at the same angle as the ear canal, rubber tubing, and a head with either a diaphragm or a bell and a diaphragm (a dual-headed stethoscope) (Figure 4-2). The bell transmits low-frequency sounds; the diaphragm accentuates high-frequency sounds. Stethoscopes are available in a variety of styles and prices. Although the choice of style (e.g., Sprague Rappaport type with dual tubing from the earpieces to the head, Littman type with a single tube to the head) depends on personal preference, the pharmacist should select a quality stethoscope and avoid the cheaper models. Higher-quality stethoscopes transmit sounds more efficiently and are more

---

TABLE 4-2 *Physical Assessment Equipment*

EQUIPMENT	PURPOSE
Flashlight	Assess pupillary reflexes; aid in the inspection of the oropharynx and skin
Ophthalmoscope	Perform funduscopic exam
Otoscope	Assess external ear and tympanic membrane
Tongue depressor	Inspect oropharynx
Watch with second hand	Assess heart and respiratory rate
Thermometer	Obtain body temperature
Stethoscope	Assess cardiovascular, pulmonary, and abdominal system
Sphygmomanometer	Obtain blood pressure
Reflex hammer	Assess neurologic function
Tuning fork	Assess neurologic function

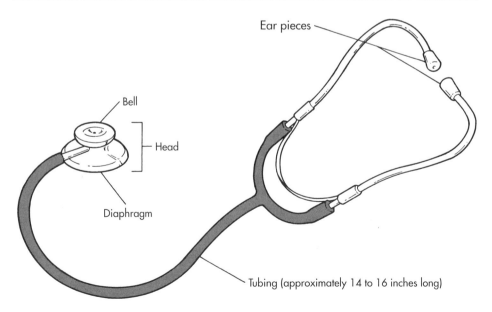

FIGURE 4-2 *The Stethoscope.* Components of the stethoscope.

durable than cheaper models. The ear pieces, which are placed in the user's ears and angled in, should fit the ear canals snugly and comfortably; the goal is for the sound to be transmitted to the eardrum through an unbroken system. Most quality stethoscopes come with several different sizes and shapes of ear tips, enabling the user to select the best fitting tips.

The ophthalmoscope consists of a head and a handle (Figure 4-3). The head contains a viewing lens control and a beam control. The viewing lens control (lens wheel) is used to focus the instrument. Positive diopters (black numbers) are used for nearsighted eyes; negative diopters (red numbers) are used for farsighted eyes. The beam control is used to select the aperture (beam). The selection of aperture depends on the structure being assessed (Table 4-3).

The otoscope consists of a head and a handle (Figure 4-4). The head, which contains a speculum and magnifying glass, can be rotated up and down in several positions. Disposable speculum covers are available in a variety of sizes to fit most ear canals. Most otoscopes and ophthalmoscopes are available as interchangeable heads that fit the same handle.

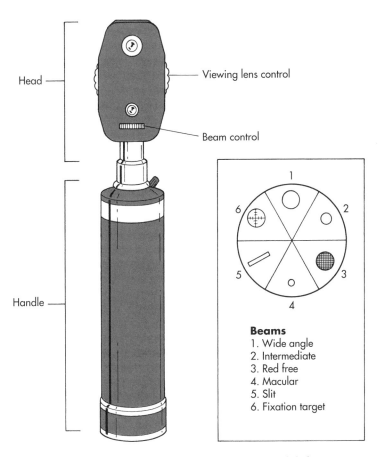

Head

Viewing lens control

Beam control

Handle

Beams
1. Wide angle
2. Intermediate
3. Red free
4. Macular
5. Slit
6. Fixation target

FIGURE **4-3** *The Ophthalmoscope.* Components of the ophthalmoscope.

TABLE 4-3	*Ophthalmoscope Apertures*
APERTURE	**USE**
Wide angle	Assess dilated pupils
Intermediate	Assess undilated pupils and details of small areas
Red free	Assess retinal vessels
Macular	Assess macula
Slit	Assess cornea, anterior chamber, and elevations or depressions in the fundus
Fixation target	Assess eccentric fixation

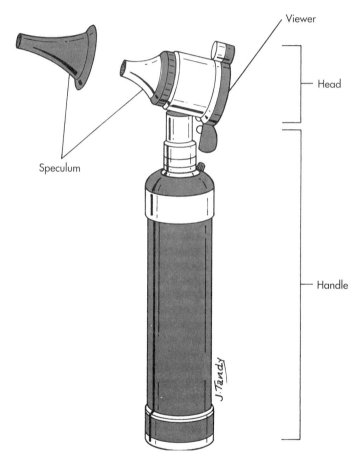

Viewer

Head

Speculum

Handle

FIGURE 4-4 *The Otoscope.* Components of the otoscope.

THE SKIN

The skin is evaluated using inspection and palpation for color (pallor, cyanosis, redness, yellowness), hydration (dry, moist), temperature (warm, cool), texture (rough, smooth), thickness (thick, thin), and mobility (immobile, mobile, hypermobile). Lesions are described according to location, type, color, shape, size, grouping, and pattern. The nails and nail beds are evaluated for clubbing, cyanosis, and trauma.

Terminology
Lesions
Primary lesions
bulla A large (>1 cm), circumscribed, elevated lesion containing serous fluid such as blistering from second-degree burns

ecchymosis A large (>1 cm) hemorrhage, commonly known as a bruise

macule A small (<1 cm), circumscribed, flat, discolored lesion such as a freckle or flat nevus

nodule A large (>1 cm), solid lesion that may be below, even with, or above the surface of the skin

papule A small (<1 cm), elevated, solid lesion such as a wart

patch An area containing discolored, circumscribed, and flat or elevated groups of lesions such as a measles rash

petechia A small (<2 mm) hemorrhage

plaque A large (>1 cm), circumscribed, elevated, and solid lesion such as pityriasis rosea

pustule A circumscribed, elevated lesion of varying size containing pus such as impetigo

vesicle A small (<1 cm), circumscribed, elevated lesion containing serous fluid such as herpes zoster

wheal An edematous and transitory papule such as hives

Secondary lesions
crust A mass of dried exudate such as impetigo

excoriation A scratch mark usually covered with blood or serous crusts

fissure A linear break in the skin

keloid A hypertrophic scar

lichenification Thickening and roughening of the skin with increased visibility of normal skin lines

scale Dead epidermal cells such as dandruff

scar Area in which normal skin tissue has been replaced by connective tissue

ulcer An irregularly sized and shaped excavation that extends below the dermal skin layer such as a pressure sore

Other lesions
comedo (blackhead) A pilosebaceous follicular plug of sebaceous and keratinous material

milium (whitehead) A small (1 to 2 mm) nodule with no visible opening.

nevus (mole) A flat or elevated pigmented lesion

Osler's node A small, raised, discolored, tender lesion on the pads of the fingers and toes associated with bacterial endocarditis

telangiectasias Dilated superficial blood vessels

Fingernail and Toenail Terms
Beau's lines Transverse horizontal depressions associated with severe illness

clubbing Increased angle (>180°) between the base of the nail and the nail bed;

associated with chronic arterial desaturation (e.g., chronic obstructive pulmonary disease [COPD])

koilonychia Spooning of the nails associated with iron deficiency anemia

onychcolysis Separation of the nail from the nail bed associated with trauma, malnutrition, and thyroid disease

splinter hemorrhages Red or brown linear streaks in the distal extremity of the nail bed; nonspecific

THE HEAD AND NECK

The structures of the head and neck are evaluated by inspection and palpation. Neck veins (see page 73) and thyroid bruits are evaluated by auscultation. The visual acuity, hearing, and facial and ophthalmic reflexes are tested when clinically indicated (see pages 65-66, 87). Assessment of the head and neck includes assessment of the skull, scalp, face, neck, nose, ears, mouth and pharynx, and eyes.

Skull

The size, contour, and shape of the skull are assessed by inspection and palpation.

Hair

The quantity, texture, and distribution of hair are assessed by inspection.

Scalp

The scalp is inspected for lesions and scales.

Face

The face is inspected for expression, symmetry, movements, lesions, and edema.

Neck

The neck is inspected for symmetry, masses, and enlargement of the parotid and submaxillary glands and lymph nodes. The sternomastoid muscles are inspected and palpated. The position of the trachea is noted and the carotid arteries assessed by inspection and auscultation. The thyroid is palpated for size, shape, symmetry, tenderness, and nodules; a bruit may be heard on auscultation if the thyroid is enlarged. The lymph nodes (Figure 4-5) are palpated for size, shape, mobility, and tenderness.

Nose

The external nose and nasal cavity are inspected for symmetry, inflammation, and lesions. The sinuses are palpated; the frontal and maxillary sinuses also may be evaluated by transillumination. Transillumination of the maxillary sinuses is performed by placing a bright light in the mouth; illuminated maxillary sinuses appear as dull crescent-shaped glowing areas under each eye. The frontal sinuses are transilluminated by placing a light source under the medial aspect of each eyebrow; the frontal sinuses appear as glowing areas above each eye.

Ears

The external ear is inspected and palpated for nodules. The ear canal and tympanic membranes are inspected with an otoscope. The otoscope is inserted by tipping the

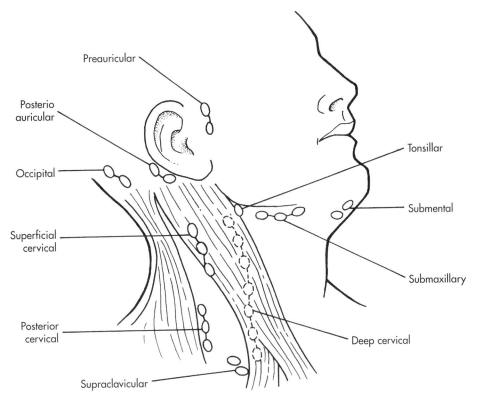

Preauricular

Posterio auricular

Occipital

Superficial cervical

Posterior cervical

Supraclavicular

Tonsillar

Submental

Submaxillary

Deep cervical

FIGURE 4-5 *Head and Neck Lymph Nodes.* Lymph nodes are located in many regions of the head and neck. (From Delp MH, Manning RT: *Major's physical diagnosis,* ed 9, Philadelphia, 1991, W.B. Saunders.)

patient's head slightly to the opposite side and gently pulling the auricle up, back, and slightly outward. (Caution: movement of the auricle and tragus is painful if the patient has acute otitis externa.) The canal is inspected for foreign bodies, discharge, color, and edema. The tympanic membrane is inspected for color, perforations, bulging, and air-fluid levels.

Hearing

A general (and relatively inaccurate) assessment of hearing is obtained by testing the ability of the patient to hear, one ear at a time, a sequence of equally accented syllables (e.g., three-five-two-four) whispered from a distance of a couple of feet. The Rinne test, which compares bone and air conduction, is performed by initially placing the end of a vibrating tuning fork (128 Hz or 512 Hz) on the mastoid process behind the ear; this tests bone conduction. The patient is instructed to signal when the sound is no longer heard. At that time the tuning fork is removed from the mastoid process and held in front of but not touching the ear canal; this tests air conduction. Normally air conduction is better than bone conduction; that is, the patient can once again hear the vibrating tuning fork when the tuning fork is placed in front of the ear canal. The Weber's test is performed by placing the end of a vibrating tuning fork on the center of the patient's forehead. Normally, the sound is heard equally well in both ears. In conduction loss the sound is heard best in the impaired ear; in unilateral sensorineural hearing loss the sound is heard best in the unimpaired ear.

Mouth and Pharynx

The lips and mucosa are inspected for color, ulcerations, hydration, and lesions. The teeth and gums are inspected for color, bleeding, inflammation, caries, missing teeth, ulcerations, and lesions. The hard palate is inspected for color, architecture, symmetry, ulcerations, and lesions. The movement of the soft palate (elevation and symmetry) is noted when the patient says "ah." The tonsils and posterior palate are inspected for color, edema, ulcerations, exudates, and lesions. The top, sides, and bottom of the tongue are inspected for color, symmetry, ulcerations, and lesions. The odor of the breath is noted (alcohol odor in alcoholic intoxication; urinous odor in uremia; sweetish fruity odor in diabetes mellitus with ketoacidosis; a musty odor [fetor hepaticus] in severe parenchymal liver disease).

Eyes

The external and internal structures of the eyes are evaluated, and if indicated visual acuity is assessed using a Snellen eye chart, the familiar chart with the large E on the top line followed by a series of lines with increasingly smaller print. A general assessment of visual acuity can be obtained by asking the patient to read any printed material (book, magazine, newspaper). The peripheral visual fields are tested by the confrontation technique, which consists of bringing a small object (usually the examiner's finger) from the patient's visual periphery into the patient's field of vision from several different directions (top, bottom, right side, left side); the examiner can stand in front of or behind the patient. The extraocular muscles are tested by having the patient follow the movements of the examiner's finger in the six cardinal directions (elevation, depression, adduction, abduction, extorsion, intorsion). The eyes normally follow the finger smoothly and in parallel with the movements; however, far lateral nystagmus may occur normally.

The position and alignment of the eyes are noted. If exophthalmos (abnormal protrusion of the eyeball) is observed, the eye should be inspected from above and the relationship of the cornea to the eyelids noted. The eyelids are inspected for color, lesions, edema, and condition of the eyelashes. The conjunctiva are inspected for color and edema. The cornea and lens are inspected for opacities. The corneal blink reflex is tested by lightly touching the cornea with a tissue; the normal reflex is to blink.

The iris and pupil are inspected for size, shape, and equality. The iris is assessed for the presence of abnormal pigments or deposits. The pupillary reaction to light is tested by briefly flicking a light on the pupil and noting the direct and consensual (opposite eye) pupillary constriction; both pupils normally constrict in response to the light stimulus. The pupillary reaction to accommodation is tested by having the patient focus on an object (usually the examiner's finger) from several feet away and then noting the pupillary constriction and convergence ("cross-eyed" response) of the eyes as the object is brought to within a few centimeters in front of the eyes.

The ophthalmoscope is used to evaluate the fundi. The appropriate light beam and diopter are selected (see page 62). The examiner's right hand and right eye are used to evaluate the patient's right eye; the left hand and left eye are used to evaluate the patient's left eye. The examiner should take a moment to focus the instrument on the wrinkles of the examiner's palm held a few inches in front of the instrument; this adjusts the ophthalmoscope to the examiner's eye and saves time adjusting to the patient's eye. The examiner should place the hand not holding the ophthalmoscope on the patient's forehead; this steadies the head and prevents the examiner and patient from bumping foreheads during the examination. If necessary, the examiner can use this hand to lift the patient's eyelid. The patient is instructed to look straight ahead. The light beam is aimed at the pupil from a distance of about 15 inches and slightly lateral to the patient's line of vision; the light beam is on target when the eye appears red-orange (the red reflex); the red-orange color is the light reflecting from the retina. The examiner moves straight toward the patient, never losing the red reflex, until the examiner's forehead touches the hand steadying the patient's head. The diopters are adjusted until the internal structures of the eye are brought into clear focus. Note that refocusing is required as different structures and areas of the retina are assessed.

The optic disc, physiologic cup, retinal blood vessels, macula, and retina are visualized with the ophthalmoscope (Figure 4-6). No set sequence is followed in visualizing these structures. The retina, the red-orange area on which the other structures are located, is inspected for the presence of lesions. The retinal blood vessels are usually the first structures seen. The retinal arteries and veins emerge from the optic disc and have the highest density in the vicinity of the optic disc. Retinal arteries are thinner and brighter red than retinal veins. The size, color, and status of the arteriovenous crossings in all regions of the eyes are assessed. The optic disc, the head of the optic nerve (also known as the blind spot), is the most obvious structure. It is a yellowish-pink ovoid 1.5 mm in diameter with sharp margins (the margins closest to the nose may be blurred). The physiologic cup, the depressed

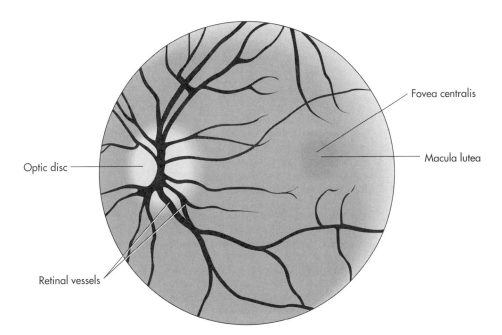

FIGURE 4-6 *Retinal Landmarks.* The retina as seen through the ophthalmoscope.

center of the optic disc, is lighter in color than the optic disc and normally occupies about one third of the diameter of the optic disc (cup-to-disc ratio). The optic disc is inspected for size, shape, and sharpness of the borders, and the cup-to-disc ratio is estimated. The macula is a small, round, and extremely light-sensitive area located about two disc-diameters temporally from the optic disc in an area nearly free of retinal blood vessels; the red-free filter is used to inspect the macula. The fovea is the slightly depressed area in the center of the macula.

Terminology

acromegaly A pituitary disorder characterized by a massive face with enlarged lower jaw, prominent nose and eyebrows, and coarse facial features

astigmatism A condition characterized by unequal curvatures of the cornea

AV nicking An abnormality visualized on funduscopic examination and associated with hypertension; at arteriovenous crossings the vein appears to stop abruptly on either side of the arteriole

AV tapering An abnormality visualized on funduscopic examination and associated with hypertension; at arteriovenous crossings the vein appears to taper off on either side of the arteriole

Bell's palsy Unilateral paralysis of the facial nerve

Chvostek's sign Contraction or spasm of the facial muscles associated with tetany and hypocalcemia; elicited by tapping the face sharply with a finger just in front of the external auditory meatus over the facial nerve

conjunctival injection Dilated conjunctival vessels

copper wires An abnormality visualized on funduscopic examination and associated with hypertension; appears as a coppery strip of light along the surface of the vessel

corneal arcus A thin, gray-white circle around the cornea; associated with aging

deep hemorrhage An abnormality visualized on funduscopic examination and associated with diabetes; appears as small, irregular red spots in the retina

exophthalmos Abnormal protrusion of the eyeball; associated with Graves' disease

fetor hepaticus A musty odor of breath associated with severe parenchymal liver disease

fissured tongue Increased tongue fissures; benign; sometimes associated with aging

flame hemorrhage An abnormality visualized on funduscopic examination; associated with hypertension; appears as small, linear hemorrhages in the retina

geographic tongue Denuded areas of papillae; benign

hairy tongue Elongated papillae; benign; associated with antibiotic therapy

hirsutism Increased hair growth in androgen-sensitive areas (e.g., beard or mustache areas); associated with ovarian, adrenal, thyroid, and pituitary disorders and some medications

hyperopia Farsightedness

Koplik's spots Small blue-white spots with red margins found on the mucous membranes near the parotid duct; associated with measles; appear before the skin lesions are visible

micoraneurysms An abnormality visualized on funduscopic examination; associated with diabetes; appear as tiny red spots in the macular area

muddy sclera Brownish sclera; benign; commonly found in dark-skinned individuals

myopia Nearsightedness

normocephalic, atraumatic A physical examination finding meaning that the head is a normal size and shape and no evidence of trauma is present *palpebral fissure* The space, when the eyes are open, between the upper and lower eyelids

periorbital edema Puffiness of the upper and lower eyelids

Rinne test A hearing test that compares air and bone conduction

smooth red tongue Finding associated with deficiencies of vitamin B_{12}, niacin, and iron

Weber's test A hearing test that compares bone conduction in both ears

xanthelasma Yellow, raised, well-circumscribed plaques found in the skin around the eyelids; associated with hypercholesterolemia

THE CHEST AND LUNGS

Assessment of the chest and lungs requires a clear understanding of the anatomic locations of the five lobes of the lung. The vertical reference points include the midsternal, midclavicular, anterior axillary, midaxillary, posterior axillary, scapular, and vertebral lines (Figure 4-7). The anterior and posterior locations of the five lobes of the lungs are different. On the anterior view the apex of the lung extends 3 to 4 cm above the medial end of the clavicles. The base of the lung extends to approximately the sixth to the eighth rib. The horizontal fissure separating the right upper and middle lobes is located from the fourth rib at the midsternal line to the fifth rib at the midaxillary line. The oblique fissure separating the right middle and lower lobes is located from the fifth rib at the midaxillary line to the sixth rib at the midclavicular line; the left oblique fissure separating the left upper and lower lobes is located at a similar position on the left. On the posterior view the right and left oblique fissures separating the right upper and lower lobes and left upper and lower lobes, respectively, are located from approximately the third thoracic vertebra medially to the sixth rib laterally. The base of the lung extends to approximately the ninth to the twelfth thoracic vertebra.

The techniques of inspection, percussion, palpation, and auscultation are used to assess the chest and lungs.

Inspection

The chest is inspected during at least one complete respiratory cycle for chest wall abnormalities, use of accessory muscles, anteroposterior diameter, and skeletal abnormalities.

Percussion

Percussion is used to assess the density of underlying lung tissue and determine the movement of the diaphragm during the respiratory cycle (diaphragmatic excursion). To percuss, the pleximeter finger is placed parallel to the ribs in the intercostal space. The character of the resulting vibrations is assessed by both sound and feel. Normally percussion produces a loud, low-pitched, resonant note. Increased air spaces, as in emphysema, produces a very loud, low-pitched, hyperresonant note. Areas of consolidation produce a dull or flat note. Shifting dullness is associated with free fluid within the pleural cavity. All lobes are assessed, and both sides are compared. The location of the diaphragm is determined with the lungs fully expanded and emptied; normal diaphragmatic movement is about 3 to 5 cm for females and 5 to 6 cm for males with the right diaphragm located slightly higher than the left. Diaphragmatic excursion is assessed by percussing posteriorly from about the sixth rib in the midscapular line downward with the lungs fully

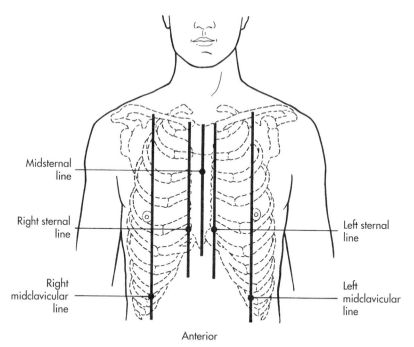

Midsternal line

Right sternal line

Left sternal line

Right midclavicular line

Left midclavicular line

Anterior

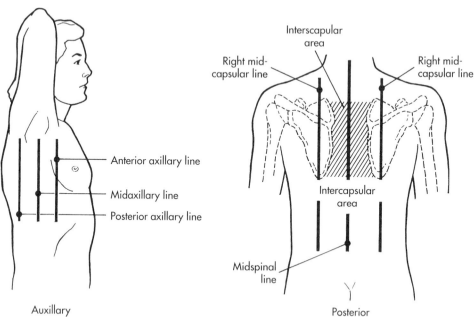

Interscapular area

Right mid-capsular line

Right mid-capsular line

Anterior axillary line

Midaxillary line

Posterior axillary line

Intercapsular area

Midspinal line

Auxillary

Posterior

FIGURE 4-7 *Thorax Topography.* Anterior, posterior, and axillary landmarks. (From Delp MH, Manning RT: *Major's physical diagnosis,* ed 9, Philadelphia, 1991, W.B. Saunders.)

expanded; the process is repeated with the lungs emptied. The diaphragm is located where the percussion note changes from resonant to dull.

Palpation

Palpation is used to locate masses, pulsations, and other abnormalities such as crepitation; identify the location of the trachea; and assess for tactile fremitus. Tactile fremitus is assessed by having the patient say "ninety-nine" or "one-two-three"; the vibrations created are felt with the palmar surfaces of the hand.

Auscultation

The lungs are auscultated using a stethoscope. The diaphragm of the stethoscope is placed flat against the chest wall and the sounds from all lung fields are assessed and compared. Breath sounds are elicited by having the patient breathe deeply and slowly through the mouth on command. One complete respiratory cycle (inspiration and expiration) should be assessed at each location. Normal breath sounds include tracheobronchial, bronchovesicular, and vesicular breath sounds. Abnormal breath sounds include wheezes, rhonchi, stridor, and crackles. A pleural friction rub may be heard when the visceral and parietal pleurae rub together. The friction rub, which sounds like squeaking leather, is heard best at the base of the lung. Voice sounds (egophony, whispered pectoriloquy) are transmitted more clearly over areas of consolidation; vocal resonance is decreased over areas of hyperinflation.

Terminology

apnea Absence of respiration

barrel chest An anteroposterior diameter ratio of 1:1; associated with diseases characterized by air trapping (e.g., COPD)

Biot's respiration Irregular respiration; may occur in meningitis

bradypnea Abnormally slow respiratory rate with regular rhythm and normal depth of breathing; associated with central nervous system depressants and elevated intracranial pressure

bronchial breath sounds Loud, high-pitched, normal breath sounds heard over the manubrium; normal inspiratory/expiratory ratio of 1:3

bronchovesicular breath sounds Normal breath sounds heard over the main stem bronchi just distal to the central airways; softer and lower pitched than tracheal breath sounds with equal inspiratory and expiratory duration and pitch

Cheyne-Stokes respiration A cyclic, abnormal respiratory pattern characterized by a gradual increase in the depth and rate of respiration followed by a gradual decrease in the depth and rate ending in apnea; characteristic of diseases that affect the central respiratory centers

consolidation Increased density

crackles Discontinuous, short-duration, bubbling sounds

crepitation Crackling

dullness or flatness Soft, medium-pitched percussion notes elicited over areas of increased density

egophony Altered vocal resonance over areas of consolidation; the spoken "e-e-e-e" is transmitted as "a-a-a-a"

eupnea Normal respiration

funnel chest (pectus excavatum) Finding in which the lower part of the sternum is depressed *hyperpnea* Increased depth and rate of respiration

hyperresonance A loud, low-pitched percussion note elicited over areas of increased air volume

Kussmaul's breathing Deep, rapid respiration; characteristic of coma and diabetic ketoacidosis

kyphoscoliosis Combined kyphosis and scoliosis

kyphosis Abnormal curvature of the spine with backward convexity

pigeon chest Anterior displacement of the sternum

pleural friction rub An abnormal, creaking, leatherlike sound produced when the inflamed surfaces of the visceral and parietal pleura rub against one another

resonance The loud, low-pitched percussion note elicited over normal lung tissue

rhonchi Coarse, rattling, abnormal breath sounds; often change location after coughing

scoliosis Abnormal lateral curvature of the spine

stridor Abnormal, high-pitched, continuous lung sounds heard over the upper airway

tachypnea Increased respiratory rate

tactile fremitus Palpable vocal vibrations felt through the chest wall; increased over areas of consolidation; decreased over obstructed areas and pleural abnormalities

tracheal breath sounds Very loud and high-pitched harsh normal breath sounds heard over the extrathoracic trachea

tracheobronchial breath sounds Loud, high-pitched, normal breath sounds heard over large bronchi; a slight pause occurs between inspiratory and expiratory sounds; inspiratory duration shorter than expiratory duration

tympany Loud, drumlike percussion notes elicited over hyperinflated areas

vesicular breath sounds Soft, low-pitched, normal breath sounds heard over peripheral lung tissue; inspiratory duration longer than expiratory duration

wheezes Abnormal, high-pitched, continuous breath sounds; associated with airway obstruction

whispered pectoriloquy Whispered voice sounds are transmitted more loudly and clearly than normal; associated with areas of cavitation and consolidation

THE CARDIOVASCULAR SYSTEM

Assessment of the chest and cardiovascular system requires a clear understanding of the anatomic position of the heart (Figure 4-8). The right ventricle occupies most of the anterior cardiac surface with the right atrium along a narrow border from the third to the fifth rib just right of the sternum; the other chambers of the heart are not normally identifiable on examination. The left ventricular apex (apical impulse or point of maximal impulse) is normally located at the intersection of the fifth intercostal space and the midclavicular line. The base of the heart is located between the right second intercostal space medial to the sternum to the left second intercostal space medial to the sternum.

The techniques of inspection, palpation, and auscultation are used to assess the heart. The examination is always conducted from the patient's right side. Although very light percussion may be used to determine the cardiac borders and assess for the presence of pericardial effusions, aortic aneurysm, and mediastinal tumors, percussion is not a part of the routine cardiovascular examination.

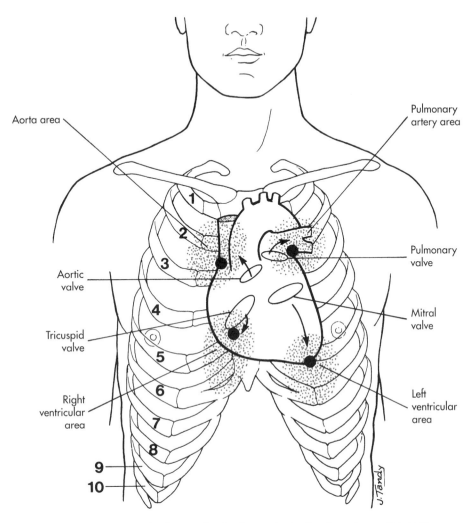

FIGURE 4-8 *Cardiovascular Topography.* Cardiovascular landmarks and auscultatory areas. (From Delp MH, Manning RT: *Major's physical diagnosis,* ed 9, Philadelphia, 1991, W.B. Saunders.)

Inspection

The chest is inspected for visible cardiac motions and the neck veins are inspected for jugular venous pressure (JVP) and waveforms. The jugular vein is located in the neck next to the point where the sternocleidomastoid muscle attaches to the clavicle. The jugular vein is inspected with the patient supine and the head of the bed elevated to 15 to 30 degrees. JVP is measured as the vertical distance between the highest point at which pulsations of the jugular vein can be seen and the sternal angle. Because JVP depends on the angle of elevation of the head, both the vertical distance and the angle of elevation of the bed are recorded. Estimation of JVP by this method is highly inaccurate. A more general assessment is that the right atrial pressures are high (>15 mmHg) when the jugular vein is distended to the jaw when the patient is seated at a 90-degree angle. The waveforms are easiest to see in the right jugular vein, which is straighter than the left. The waveform of the jugular vein is assessed by observation (Figure 4-9). The *a* wave results from atrial contraction. The *v* wave results from the pressures transmitted just before the opening of the tricuspid valve. The *x* descent follows the *a* wave and represents decreased pressure as blood flows into the atrium. The *y* descent follows the *v* wave and represents decreased pressure as blood flows into the ventricle. Normally only the *a* and *v* waves are visible.

Palpation

Chest wall palpation is used to locate the point of maximal impulse (PMI) and assess local and general cardiac motion and cardiac thrills. With the patient sitting the clinician locates the PMI with the fingertips. The PMI has a normal diameter of about 2 to 3 cm and is normally located within 10 cm of the midsternal line. Local and general cardiac motion is assessed with the fingertips; the patient is in a supine position. Pericardial friction rubs and thrills may be palpable. A small stick or straw may be used to amplify the motion.

The cardiovascular examination includes assessment of the peripheral pulses. The peripheral arterial pulses include the radial, carotid, brachial, femoral, popliteal, posterior tibial, and dorsalis pedis pulses (Figure 4-10). Pulses are rated as normal, diminished, or absent; a rating scale may be used. The typical rating scale uses 4+ to denote the normal pulse, with 3+, 2+, 1+, and 0 representing progressive degrees of diminishment (Table 4-4). The cardiac rate and rhythm are assessed by palpating the radial pulse.

Table 4-4	*Peripheral Vascular Pulse Rating Scale*		
RATING	**MEANING**	**RATING**	**MEANING**
0	Completely absent pulses	3+	Slightly impaired pulses
1+	Markedly impaired pulses	4+	Normal pulses
2+	Moderately impaired pulses		

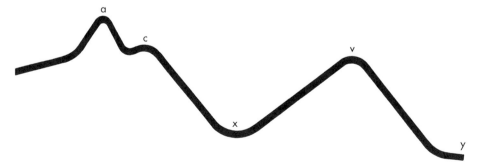

FIGURE 4-9 *Jugular Venous Waveforms.* The jugular venous waveforms vary with atrial pressures. *a*, Atrial contraction; *c*, bulging of tricuspid valve into the right atrium; *x*, decreased pressures as blood flows into the atrium; *v*, pressure increased just before tricuspid valve opens; *y*, decreased pressure as blood flows into the ventricle.

Auscultation

Auscultation follows inspection and palpation; the stethoscope is applied directly to the skin. The diaphragm, used to assess higher-pitched sounds, is applied tightly to the skin. The bell, used to assess lower-pitched sounds, is applied loosely to the skin. A great deal of practice and experience is required to identify and distinguish

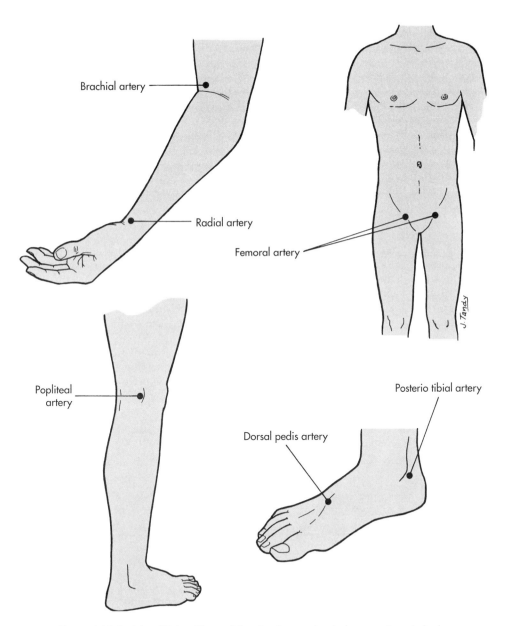

FIGURE 4-10 *Peripheral Pulses.* The peripheral pulses are located over major arteries in the upper extremities, inguinal area, and lower extremities.

among the variety of normal and abnormal heart sounds. Heart sounds are very soft; listening in a quiet area or closing the eyes may be helpful.

The four auscultatory areas are identified in Figure 4-8. They are close to but not the same as the anatomic locations of the valves. The aortic auscultatory area is located over the second intercostal space at the right sternal border, the pulmonic auscultatory area is located over the second intercostal space at the left sternal border, the tricuspid auscultatory area is located over the left lower sternal border, and the mitral auscultatory area is located at the cardiac apex (fifth intercostal space midclavicular line).

The first heart sound (S_1), created by mitral and tricuspid valve closure, is loudest at the cardiac apex. The second heart sound (S_2), created by aortic and pulmonic valve closure, is loudest at the base. The second heart sound can be "split" into the aortic and pulmonic components by deep inspiration (physiologic splitting) or disease (e.g., pulmonary hypertension). The third heart sound (S_3), an abnormal heart sound associated with volume overload, is a soft sound heard just after S_2. The fourth heart sound (S_4), an abnormal heart sound associated with pressure overload, is a soft sound heard just before S_1. S_1 and S_2 are assessed in all four auscultatory areas with the patient in the upright and supine positions. The relationship of breathing to the intensity of the cardiac sounds should be noted. Palpation of the carotid helps determine the timing of cardiac events and sounds (the S_1 precedes and the S_2 follows the carotid pulse).

Other abnormal heart sounds include opening snaps (associated with mitral stenosis), ejection clicks (associated with sudden dilation of the aorta and the pulmonary artery), and midsystolic clicks (associated with floppy mitral valves). Gallops are exaggerated normal diastolic sounds; friction rubs are associated with pericarditis. Some heart sounds are heard best if the patient is in a specific body position. For example, aortic sounds and pericardial friction rubs are heard best when the patient sits up and leans forward. S_3 and S_4 and the murmurs of aortic insufficiency and mitral stenosis are heard best when the patient is supine and turned to the left.

Murmurs are abnormal heart sounds created by turbulent flow across a valve or the septum and by functional defects such as anemia and hyperthyroidism. Murmurs are described according to their timing in the cardiac cycle (systolic murmurs occur between S_1 and S_2; diastolic murmurs occur between S_2 and S_1), loudest location, radiation, shape of the sound (crescendo, decrescendo, crescendo-decrescendo, continuous), duration (continuous; early-, mid-, late-systolic; diastolic; holosystolic; pansystolic), intensity (grade I through VI) (Table 4-5), and

Table 4-5	*Murmur Rating Scale*
GRADE	**MEANING**
I	Very faint
II	Soft
III	Moderately loud
IV	Loud
V	Very loud; may be heard with the stethoscope partially off the chest wall
VI	Very loud; can be head with the stethoscope off the chest wall

pitch or quality of sound (low, medium, high). A palpable murmur is known as a *thrill.*

Auscultation also is used to detect vascular murmurs, known as *bruits.* Bruits, sounds made by turbulent blood flow, are heard over vessels with constricted lumens. The carotid and femoral arteries are routinely assessed for bruits; bruits are sometimes found over the vertebral, subclavian, and abdominal arteries.

Blood Pressure

The peripheral blood pressure is measured using a blood pressure cuff, mercury or aneroid sphygmomanometer, and stethoscope. Both types of sphygmomanometers are accurate and easy to use; however, the mercury column must be kept vertical and the numbers read at eye level with the meniscus. Aneroid sphygmomanometers must be recalibrated periodically.

Appropriately sized cuffs must be used; falsely elevated pressures result from using cuffs that are too short or narrow. The bag width should be about 40% of the limb circumference with the bag length about 80% of the limb circumference. The cuff must be positioned appropriately. The arterial portion of the cuff is placed directly over the brachial artery with the bottom of the edge approximately 2.5 cm above the antecubital crease (Figure 4-11). The location of the brachial artery should be identified by palpation before the cuff is placed on the limb. The patient's arm should be supported at the level of the heart; tensed muscles falsely elevate the blood pressure. To obtain the blood pressure, place the stethoscope over the brachial artery and inflate the cuff to about 20 to 30 mmHg over the predicted or known systolic blood pressure. The cuff is deflated at approximately 3 mmHg per second. The systolic blood pressure is the pressure at which at least two beats are audible. As the pressure falls, the beats become louder and then slowly diminish before disappearing altogether. The diastolic pressure is the pressure at which the beats are no longer audible. Depending on the clinical situation, the blood pressure may need to be obtained in both arms and in more than one body position (i.e., sitting and standing, sitting and supine). Repetitive reinflation of the cuff after partial deflation causes venous congestion and inaccurate blood pressure assessments.

Terminology

bradycardia A slow (<50 beats per minute) heart rate

bruit An abnormal auscultatory sound heard over a blood vessel; associated with turbulent blood flow

crescendo, decrescendo murmur A murmur that increases and then decreases in intensity

diastolic murmur A murmur heard during diastole

ejection clicks Abnormal heart sounds caused by dilation of the aortic and pulmonary arteries

gallop rhythms Exaggerated diastolic heart sounds

holosystolic murmur A murmur heard throughout systole

hypertension Elevated blood pressure

hypotension Low blood pressure

midsystolic clicks Abnormal heart sounds caused by floppy mitral valves

opening snap An abnormal diastolic heart sound caused by the opening of a stenotic mitral valve

orthostatic hypotension A fall in systolic blood pressure of 15 mmHg or more when the patient assumes a more upright position

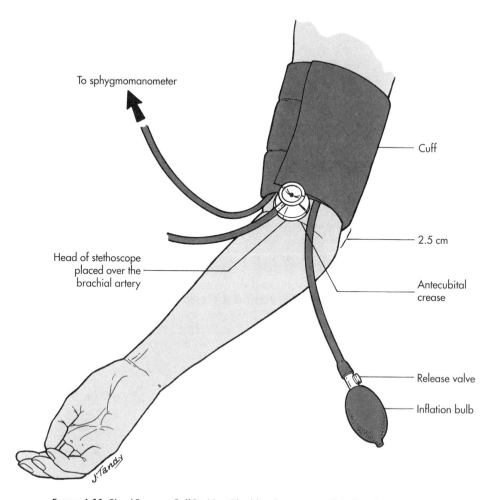

FIGURE 4-11 *Blood Pressure Cuff Position.* The blood pressure cuff and stethoscope must be positioned correctly in order to obtain an accurate assessment of the blood pressure.

pansystolic murmur A murmur heard throughout systole

pericardial friction rub An abnormal sound created when the visceral and parietal pericardial membranes rub against one another

point of maximal impulse (PMI) Right ventricular thrust (apical impulse)

pulsus alternans Regular alteration of high and low pulse beats; associated with heart failure

pulsus paradoxus Decreased systolic blood pressure with inspiration; normally about 5 mmHg

regurgitant murmur A murmur produced by backflow of blood across an incompetent valve

S_1 The first heart sound; produced by mitral and tricuspid valve closure

S_2 The second heart sound; produced by aortic and pulmonic valve closure

S_3 The third heart sound; produced by the sudden distension of the ventricular wall during ventricular filling; associated with heart failure

S_4 The fourth heart sound; produced by increased left ventricular end diastolic pressure and loss of ventricular distensibility; associated with hypertension

split S_2 Finding in which both components of the second heart sound (aortic and pulmonic) are distinguishable; may result from deep inspiration and any disease that delays the closure of the pulmonic valve

stenosis murmur A murmur produced by the pathologic narrowing of the orifice of a valve

systolic ejection murmur A murmur caused by increased flow across a normal valve, valvular or subvalvular stenosis, or other deformity of the valve

systolic murmur A murmur heard during systole

tachycardia A rapid (>100 beats per minute) heart rate

thrill Palpable vibrations produced by turbulent blood flow

BREASTS AND AXILLAE

The breasts are evaluated with the patient in sitting and supine positions. The breasts are inspected for size, symmetry, contour, and appearance of the skin. Abnormal findings on inspection include visible masses, dimpling, localized flattening, rashes, ulcers, and discharge from the nipple. The breasts are palpated for nodules, indurations, and areas of tenderness or increased warmth. The axillary lymph nodes, including the pectoral, subscapular, and lateral groups, are located high in the axilla close to the ribs. These nodes are palpated for size, consistency, and tenderness.

Terminology

gynecomastia Hypertrophy of breast tissue; associated with liver cirrhosis, Addison's disease, Klinefelter's syndrome, and some medications (e.g., spironolactone)

mastodynia Painful breasts

peau d'orange Breast skin with an orange peel appearance (prominent pores); indicates lymphatic obstruction and is an important sign of malignancy

retraction Dimpling of the skin, nipple retraction or inversion

THE ABDOMEN

The abdominal area is divided into four quadrants (right upper, right lower, left upper, left lower) by imaginary vertical and horizontal lines that cross at the umbilicus (Figure 4-12); findings are reported by quadrant (e.g., right upper quadrant tenderness). The examination is conducted at the patient's right side with the patient supine. Although the techniques of inspection, palpation, percussion, and auscultation are used to examine the abdomen, auscultation is performed before percussion and palpation; palpation is performed last. This sequence avoids acute examination-induced changes. The patient should bend the knees and place the feet flat on the examining table if the abdomen is tense. To decrease the sensitivity of ticklish patients, have them place their hands over and guide the hand touching the abdomen.

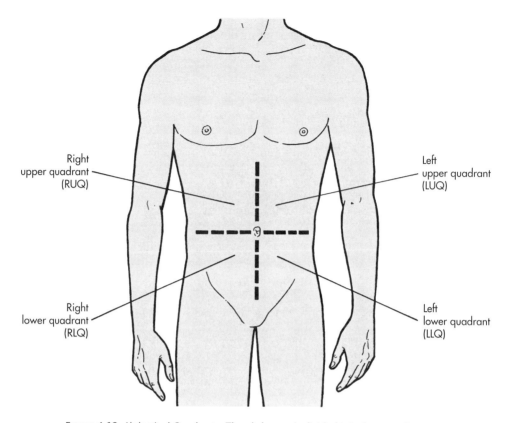

FIGURE 4-12 *Abdominal Quadrants.* The abdomen is divided into four quadrants.

Inspection

The abdomen is inspected to assess the appearance of the skin, umbilicus, and abdominal contours (scaphoid, protuberant) and note visible aortic and hepatic pulsations, peristaltic waves, and fluid shifts. Free fluid in the peritoneal cavity may shift with position, causing bulging at the flanks when the patient is supine.

Auscultation

Auscultation is used to asses bowel motility and detect abdominal bruits. Bowel sounds, produced by the mixing of fluid and air in the bowel, vary from low rumbles in loosely stretched intestines to high pitched tinkling sounds (borborygmi) in tightly stretched intestines. Bowel sounds are present with normal peristaltic movement but are absent if no peristalsis is occurring. Normal bowel sounds occur approximately every 10 seconds; auscultate for 2 minutes if normal bowel sounds are present and 3 minutes if bowel sounds are absent. Bruits may be heard over the aorta, right and left renal arteries, the right and left iliac arteries, and the right and left femoral arteries; friction rubs may be heard over the liver and spleen.

Percussion

Percussion is used to determine the liver span and differentiate between abdominal fluid and air. Percussion over the liver produces a dull note; percussion over air-filled loops of bowel produces a hollow tympanic note. The normal liver span along the right midclavicular line is about 10 cm. The liver span is determined by percussing down the midclavicular line starting at midchest. The liver span is evident as the percussion note changes from the resonant lung note to a dull liver note to a tympanic colonic note.

Areas of shifting dullness indicate freely moving fluid. Air-filled loops of bowel float to the surface of the abdomen and may obscure abdominal fluid. In these cases, a puddle sign is elicited by having the patient lie supine on the abdomen for a few moments and then shift to hands and knees. The fluid collects, or puddles, over the gravity-dependent portion of the abdomen and can be identified by percussion.

Palpation

Light palpation is used to detect areas of tenderness and rigidity. Deep palpation is used to determine the outlines of the abdominal organs and assess the size, shape, mobility, and tenderness of the lymph nodes. All four quadrants are assessed. Light palpation is performed using the pads of the fingertips and light pressure (as if kneading bread dough); deep palpation requires significant downward pressure.

The liver edge is palpated on deep inspiration just below the right costal margin. To palpate the liver, place the left hand at the posterior twelfth rib along the iliac crest and the right hand in the right upper quadrant parallel and lateral to the rectus muscle and a couple of inches below the lower margin of dullness as identified on percussion. Instruct the patient to take a deep breath and hold the breath. Lift the left hand upward and push the right hand inward and upward as the patient inspires. The liver edge, normally smooth, firm, and regular, can be felt sliding over the fingertips.

The kidneys may be palpable on deep palpation but the normal sized spleen cannot be felt on palpation; the normal duodenum and pancreas are too posterior to be palpated. The tip of an enlarged spleen may be palpated near the left tenth rib just posterior to the midaxillary line. The intraabdominal organs may not be palpable if the abdomen is obese or distended by fluid. Abdominal rigidity (tensing of the abdominal muscles) may be present if the abdomen is tender. Rebound tenderness may be elicited if the parietal peritoneum is inflamed.

A fluid wave may be elicited in patients with abdominal ascites. The fluid wave is generated by pressing the ulnar surface of one hand midline against the surface of the abdomen (this dampens the transmission of the wave through the fat layer) and then sharply tapping the lateral wall of the abdomen with the other hand. The fluid wave is transmitted to the other side of the abdomen and felt by the hand placed on the opposite lateral abdominal wall.

Terminology

ascites Free fluid in the peritoneal cavity

borborygmi Very loud gurgling and tinkling bowel sounds audible without a stethoscope; associated with hyperperistalsis

caput medusa Dilated veins radiating from the umbilicus; associated with portal vein obstruction

costal margin The edge of the lower rib cage

costovertebral angle The angle formed by the intersection of the rib cage and the vertebral column

epigastric region The upper central abdominal area

fluid wave Associated with free fluid in the abdominal cavity

hypogastric region The lower central abdominal area

peristalsis The circular intestinal contractions that propel the intestinal contents forward

puddle sign Gravity-dependent pooling of fluid at the surface of the abdomen

rebound tenderness Pain elicited when abdominal hand pressure is abruptly removed; associated with parietal peritoneal membrane inflammation

Rovsing's sign Right lower quadrant pain elicited by left-sided abdominal pressure; associated with appendicitis

scaphoid Concave-appearing abdomen

shifting dullness Dull percussion notes that shift as the patient shifts position; associated with free fluid in the abdominal cavity

spider telangiectasia (spider angioma) Dilated small surface arteries that appear as small red spots with multiple radiating arms; associated with portal hypertension

striae Discolored stripes of skin that result from ruptured elastic fibers; striae are pinkish or bluish when relatively new and more whitish when older

suprapubic region The abdominal area just above the pubic arch

umbilical region The area around the umbilicus

THE GENITOURINARY SYSTEM

The sacrococcygeal and perianal areas are inspected for the presence of lumps, ulcerations, rashes, swelling, external hemorrhoids, and excoriations. The female external genitalia (mons pubis, labia, perineum, labia minora, clitoris, urethral orifice, and introitus) are inspected for abnormalities, including lumps, ulcerations, rashes, swelling, excoriations, and discharge. The male external genitalia (penis and scrotum) are inspected for contour and abnormalities, including lumps, ulcerations, inflammation, excoriations, and swelling.

The anus and rectal wall are palpated for tone and tenderness. The prostate is palpated for size, consistency, and tenderness. The penis is palpated for indurations or other abnormalities. The structures of the scrotum (testis and epididymis) are palpated for size, shape, consistency, and tenderness. The inguinal and femoral areas are palpated for bulges that may be indicative of hernias.

The female pelvic examination consists of an inspection of the vaginal wall and cervix for color, lesions, and the shape of the cervix and cervical os. The position of the cervix is noted and cervical cells collected for cytologic evaluation (the Papanicolaou [Pap] smear). The uterus and ovaries are palpated for size, shape, consistency, masses, tenderness, and mobility. The bimanual examination is performed by palpating the internal structures between a hand placed on the abdominal wall and a finger placed in the vagina. The combined rectovaginal examination is performed by palpating the adnexa, cul-de-sac, and the uterosacral ligaments between a finger placed in the vagina and a finger placed in the rectum.

Terminology

angiokeratoma Red, slightly raised, pinpoint benign scrotal lesions; common after 50 years

anteverted, anteflexed uterus Normal uterine position

chancre A hard infectious venereal ulcer

chancroid A soft infectious venereal ulcer

condylomata acuminate Venereal warts

gravid Pregnant

hernia Protrusion of an organ through the muscular wall that normally contains the organ

hydrocele Serous fluid–containing cavity

Papanicolaou (Pap) smear Screening technique for cervical carcinoma

prostatic hypertrophy Enlarged prostate

varicocele Enlarged spermatic cord

THE MUSCULOSKELETAL SYSTEM

The structure and function of the musculoskeletal system are evaluated primarily by inspection and palpation. The curvature of the spine is noted. The musculoskeletal system is inspected for symmetry, proportion, and muscular development. The gait, stance, and ability to stand, sit, rise from a sitting position, and grasp objects are observed.

The large and small joints are assessed for range of motion. Decreased range of motion is associated with arthritis, fibrosis in or around the joint, tissue inflammation around the joint, and fixed (immobile) joints. Increased range of motion indicates increased joint mobility and may be a sign of joint instability. Limits or extension of the range of motion of a joint are reported in degrees.

Joint tenderness is assessed by gentle palpation in and around the joint. The areas in and around the joints are assessed for abnormalities such as warmth, tenderness, crepitation, and deformities. The muscles are palpated and assessed for symmetry.

Terminology

activities of daily living (ADLs) Routine activities such as getting dressed, cleaning the teeth, combing or brushing the hair, bathing, and feeding oneself

boutonnière deformity A deformity that causes flexion of the proximal interphalangeal joint with hyperextension of the distal interphalangeal joint

crepitation Audible or palpable crackling sounds

dorsiflexion Inward flexion

eversion The turning of the toes onto the great toe

extension The bending of a joint to bring the joint parallel to the long axis

flexion The bending of a joint to bring the parts of the joint into close approximation

gait The way a person walks

inversion The turning of the toes onto the small toes

kyphosis Convex backward spinal curvature

list Lateral deviation of the spine

lordosis Anteroposterior curvature of the spine (i.e., an accentuation of the normal lumbar curve)

neutral range of motion Zero degrees

plantar flexion Downward flexion of the foot

radial deviation Deviation of the fingers toward the radial bone

rheumatoid nodules Firm, nontender, unattached subcutaneous nodules at pressure points on the extensor surface of the ulna.; associated with rheumatoid arthritis

scoliosis Lateral curvature of the spine

station The way a person stands

ulnar deviation Deviation of the fingers toward the ulnar bone

THE NEUROLOGIC SYSTEM ▌

The neurologic examination consists of an assessment of mental status, the cranial nerves, sensory and motor function, cerebellar function, and reflexes. The examination is commonly limited to a simple screening examination; however, if abnormalities are suspected or detected, a complete examination is conducted.

Mental Status

Mental status is evaluated by assessing the level of consciousness (awake, alert, confused, unresponsive), orientation (to person, place, and time), affect (appropriate or inappropriate to the situation), speech and vocabulary, short- and long-term memory, judgment, abstract thinking, ability to calculate, object recognition, and praxis. Speech is assessed by having the patient say "no ifs, ands, or buts"; vocabulary is noted throughout the interview and by having the patient define a series of increasingly difficult words. Short-term memory is assessed by giving the patient three words to remember and then asking the patient to recall the words a few minutes later. Long-term memory is assessed by asking the patient about an age-appropriate, well-known past event (e.g., D day, the assassination of President Kennedy, the Challenger explosion). Judgment is assessed by asking the patient to interpret a simple problem such as "What would you do if you noticed an addressed envelope with an uncanceled stamp on the sidewalk near a mailbox?" Abstract thinking is assessed by asking the patient to interpret a common proverb such as "A bird in hand is worth two in the bush." The ability to calculate is assessed by asking the patient to perform serial seven subtractions starting at 100 (i.e., 100, 93, 86, 79). Object recognition is assessed by showing the patient several well-known objects (watch, belt, ring, tie) and asking the patient to identify the object. Praxis is assessed by asking the patient to perform a multistep motor activity such as drawing the face of a clock with a specified time.

The Cranial Nerves

The twelve cranial nerves (Table 4-6) are evaluated by assessing their function.

I—The Olfactory Nerve

The olfactory nerve is tested only if the patient complains of loss of the sense of smell or has a head injury. The olfactory nerve is tested by having the patient, with eyes closed, identify, one nostril at a time, a familiar odor (e.g., soap, coffee, toothpaste).

II–The Optic Nerve

The optic nerve is evaluated by checking the visual fields and the patient's ability to discriminate colors.

III, IV, and VI—The Oculomotor, Trochlear, and Abducens Nerves

These nerves, known collectively as the *ocular nerves*, are evaluated as a group by observing the size and shape of the pupils, pupillary reaction to light and accommodation, and extraocular movements.

V—The Trigeminal Nerve

The trigeminal nerve is evaluated by observing the patient's ability to clench the teeth and sense sharp and dull stimuli and hot and cold stimuli over the front half of the head.

VII—The Facial Nerve

The facial nerve is evaluated by observing facial movements when the patient frowns, smiles, puffs out the cheeks, whistles, and raises the eyebrows. The sensory

Table 4-6	*The Cranial Nerves*
CRANIAL NERVE	**FUNCTION**
I Olfactory	Sense of smell
II Optic	Vision
III Oculomotor	Pupillary constriction; upper eyelid elevation; most extraocular movement
IV Trochlear	Downward and inward eye movements
V Trigeminal	Temporal and masseter muscles; lateral movement of the jaw
VI Abducens	Lateral deviation of the eye
VII Facial	Facial muscle movements; sense of taste on anterior two thirds of the tongue
VIII Acoustic	Hearing and balance
IX Glossopharyngeal	Sensation of the posterior position of the eardrum, ear canal, pharynx, and posterior tongue, including taste; motor activity of the pharynx
X Vagus	Sensation of the pharynx and larynx; motor function of the palate, pharynx, and larynx
XI Accessory	Motor function of the sternomastoid and upper portion of the trapezius muscle
XII Hypoglossal	Motor activity of the tongue

function of the nerve is evaluated by assessing the patient's ability to identify sweet, sour, and salty solutions placed on the sides of the tongue.

VIII—The Acoustic Nerve

The acoustic nerve is evaluated by hearing and balance tests.

IX and X—The Glossopharyngeal and Vagus Nerves

These nerves are evaluated together by assessing the quality of speech, testing the gag reflex, and observing the movement of the soft palate and uvula.

XI—The Accessory Nerve

The accessory nerve is evaluated by observing the patient shrug the shoulders and turn the chin from side to side against resistance.

XII—The Hypoglossal Nerve

The hypoglossal nerve is evaluated by observing the patient stick out the tongue. Any fasciculations, asymmetry, deviations, and atrophy are noted.

Sensory and Motor Function

Sensory function is assessed by testing a variety of stimuli distally and working upward; the patient, with eyes closed, is asked to identify when and where the touch occurred. The stimuli include light touch (wisp of gauze or fiber), pain (sharp object such as the broken end of a tongue depressor), and vibration (vibrating tuning fork placed over a bony prominence). The major peripheral nerves and dermatomes are tested and results are compared from side to side symmetrically. Tactile localization; proprioception; and discriminative sensations such as two-point discrimination, stereognosis, graphesthesia, and point localization also are assessed.

The muscles are observed for the presence of abnormal involuntary movements, resting tone, and strength against resistance. Muscle strength on abduction and adduction is evaluated using a plus scale with zero representing no muscle contraction (complete paralysis) and five representing normal muscle strength (Table

4-7). Motor function is evaluated by assessing muscle tone during passive flexion and extension (increased resistance, normal, decreased resistance). A thorough examination includes assessment of all muscle groups in both the upper and lower extremities.

Cerebellar Function

Cerebellar function is assessed using the finger-to-nose test, the heel-to-shin test, rapid alternating movements, and the Romberg test; gait is observed. For the finger-to-nose test the examiner's finger is held at about an arm's length in front of the patient; the patient is asked to quickly and repeatedly touch the nose and then the examiner's finger. The heel-to-shin test is performed by instructing the patient to rub the heel down the shin. The rapid alternating movements test is performed by instructing the patient to pronate and supinate the hands rapidly on the thighs. The Romberg test is performed by instructing the patient to stand with the feet together, arms extended with palms up, and eyes closed. Patients with normal posterior column function can maintain the position without moving their feet for balance. Gait is assessed by observing the patient walk away, turn, and return. The patient is instructed to walk straight ahead, turn, return walking on tiptoes, turn, walk away on the heels, turn, and return walking heel-to-toe.

Reflexes

The reflexes are tested by evaluating physiologic and pathologic reflexes. Each physiologic reflex tests a different level of spinal cord function. The deep tendon (stretch) reflexes routinely tested include the biceps reflex (C5 and C6), the triceps reflex (C6 to C8), the brachioradialis reflex (C5 and C6), the patellar reflex (L2 to L4), and the Achilles reflex (S1 and S2). The abdominal reflex is a commonly tested superficial reflex. During reflex testing the patient is asked to relax the area being tested. The deep tendon reflexes are tested by striking the tendon briskly with a reflex hammer; the pointed end of the triangular head of the reflex hammer is generally used. The results are reported using a plus scale (Table 4-8), with 0 representing complete absence of the reflex, 2+ representing a normal response, and 4+ representing marked hyperreactivity. The abdominal reflex is tested by stroking each side of the abdomen above the level of the umbilicus (T8 to T10) and below the level of the umbilicus (T10 to T12); the muscles normally reflexively tighten. The plantar reflex is tested by stroking the lateral aspect of the sole of the foot from the heel to the ball of the foot with a moderately sharp object such as the handle of the reflex hammer. The normal response is for the toes to curl downward. Reflex

Table 4-7	*Muscle Strength Scale*
SCALE	MEANING
0	No muscle contractility (complete paralysis)
1+	Barely detectable contractility
2+	Active muscle contractility; unable to work against gravity
3+	Active muscle contractility; able to work against gravity but not against resistance
4+	Active muscle contractility; able to work against gravity and some resistance
5+	Active muscle contractility; able to work against gravity and full resistance (normal)

test results are frequently documented using a stick figure representation (Figure 4-13).

A variety of pathologic reflexes are associated with neurologic disease (Table 4-9). The plantar reflex is tested by stroking the bottom of the foot. A positive response, known as Babinski's reflex or sign and indicative of upper motor neuron disease, is characterized by dorsiflexion of the great toe and spreading of the other four toes. The snout, grasp, and sucking reflexes are normally present in infancy but indicate neurologic abnormalities after infancy. The snout reflex is elicited by gently tapping the patient's face just above or below the lips. A positive response is characterized by puckering of the lips. The grasp reflex is elicited by gently stroking the palm of the hand between the thumb and fingers; a positive response is characterized by flexion of the fingers. The sucking reflex is elicited by gently stroking the patient's lips from side to center with a tongue depressor. A positive response is indicated by sucking movements. Hoffmann's reflex is elicited by dorsiflexing the patient's wrist with the fingers flexed and flicking the middle finger. A positive response is characterized by adduction of the thumb or index finger. The oculocephalic reflex, also known as the *doll's eye test*, is elicited by turning the patient's head quickly from side to side. If the brainstem is intact, the eyes move in the opposite direction and maintain the straight ahead gaze position. If the brainstem is not intact, the eyes move in the direction the head is turned. The oculovestibular reflex also tests brain function. The reflex is elicited by elevating the patient's head about 30 degrees and then instilling cold water in the ear canal. If the brainstem is intact, the normal neurologic response is the development of nystagmus.

Terminology

abstract reasoning The ability to think beyond concrete terms
affect The observed emotion
anosmia Complete loss of the sense of smell

Table 4-8   *Reflex Rating Scale*

SCALE	MEANING	SCALE	MEANING
0	No response	3+	Increased response
1+	Diminished response	4+	Hyperreactive; often associated
2+	Normal physiologic response		with clonus

Table 4-9   *Reflexes Indicative of Neurologic Pathology*

REFLEX	SIGNIFICANCE	REFLEX	SIGNIFICANCE
Babinski's (plantar)	Extrapyramidal tract pathology	Hoffmann's	Corticospinal tract dysfunction
Snout	Diffuse brain disease	Oculocephalic	Brainstem pathology
Sucking	Diffuse brain disease	Oculovestibular	Brainstem pathology
Grasp	Prefrontal lobe lesions		

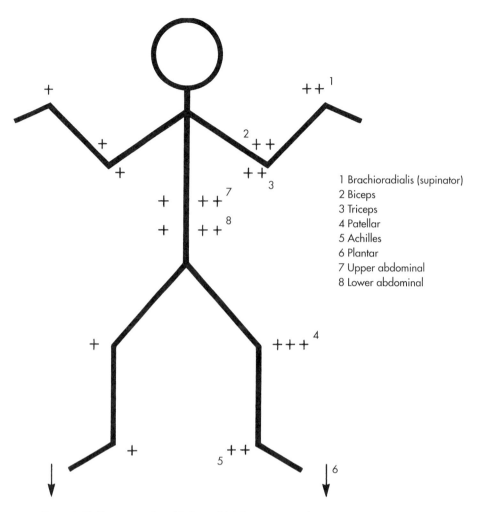

FIGURE 4-13 *Documentation of Reflexes.* Stick figures are used to document the reflexes. The pluses, indicative of the briskness of the response, are placed close to the position of the reflex. The downgoing arrows indicate normal downgoing toes.

aphasia The inability to speak

aphonia The loss of voice

asterixis Involuntary movements characterized by nonrhythmic flapping of the extremities

athetosis Involuntary movements characterized by slow, twisting irregular motions

attention The ability to focus on one activity

blocking An abnormal thought process characterized by sudden interruption of speech in midsentence

chorea Involuntary movement characterized by brief, rapid, irregular, jerky motions

circumstantiality An abnormal thought process characterized by unnecessary detail that delays reaching the point of the thought

clanging An abnormal thought process characterized by the use of words on the basis of sound instead of meaning

clonus Rhythmic oscillation between extension and flexion

coma An altered state of consciousness characterized by complete loss of consciousness, unresponsiveness to stimuli, and absence of voluntary movement

confabulation An abnormal thought process characterized by fabrication of facts or events to fill gaps in the memory

confusion An abnormality of consciousness characterized by mental slowness, inattentiveness, and incoherent thought patterns

decerebrate rigidity An abnormal body position observed in comatose patients characterized by clenched jaws, extension of the neck and legs, adduction of the arms, pronation of the forearms, and flexion of the wrists and fingers

decorticate rigidity An abnormal body position observed in comatose patients characterized by flexion of the fingers and wrists and extension and internal rotation of the legs

delirium An abnormality of consciousness characterized by confusion, agitation, and hallucinations

dysarthria Poorly coordinated, irregular speech

dyscalculia Difficulty calculating

dysgraphia Difficulty writing

dyslexia Difficulty reading

dysphasia Hesitancy and error in choosing words when speaking

dysphonia Hoarseness

dyspraxia Difficulty coordinating body movements

dystaxia Difficulty with muscle coordination

dystonia Abnormal slow, twisting, irregular movements

echolalia An abnormal thought process characterized by repetition of words or phrases spoken by others

fasciculations Involuntary movements characterized by fine twitching that rarely moves a joint

flight of ideas An abnormal thought process characterized by an almost continuous flow of accelerated speech with quick changes of subject

hemianopsia A visual field defect associated with disorders of the optic chiasm or tract

hemiplegia Paralysis of one side of the body

incoherence An abnormal thought process characterized by illogical connections and quick changes of subject

intention tremor Involuntary movements characterized by tremors that are absent at rest but appear with intentional movement

judgment The ability to compare and evaluate alternatives

loose associations Abnormal thought processes characterized by repeated shifting to unrelated subjects

mood The sustained emotional state

myoclonus Involuntary movements characterized by sudden, brief, unpredictable jerks

neologism An abnormal thought process characterized by the use of invented words or the use of words with new meanings

nystagmus Involuntary oscillation of the eyeball; described as lateral if the eyeball oscillates from side to side, vertical if the eyeball oscillates up and down, and rotatory if the eyeball oscillates in a circle

ophthalmoplegias Optic movement disorders

paraparesis A slight degree of lower extremity paralysis

paraplegia Paralysis of the lower extremities and trunk

perseveration An abnormal thought process characterized by persistent repetition of words or phrases

postural tremor Involuntary tremor that occurs when the affected part maintains position

quadriplegia Paralysis of the upper and lower extremities

recent memory Memory of information of a few hours or days

remote memory Memory of information from the distant past

resting or static tremor Involuntary movement at rest

scotoma A visual field defect associated with disorders of the optic nerve

stereognosis The ability to identity, by touch, small objects placed in the hand

stupor An abnormal state of consciousness characterized by reduced mental and physical activity and response to stimuli

thought content What a person thinks about

tics Involuntary movements characterized by brief, repetitive movements at irregular intervals

| SELF-ASSESSMENT QUESTIONS |

1 Which one of the following abbreviation/interpretation pairs is INCORRECT?
   a. A&P—auscultation and percussion
   b. NCAT—normocephalic atraumatic
   c. RRR—regular rate and rhythm
   d. CTA—clear to auscultation
   e. MSE—minor system examination

2 The term *hyperopia* means which of the following?
   a. Nearsightedness
   b. Increased intraocular pressure
   c. Farsightedness
   d. Astigmatism
   e. Abnormal protrusion of the eyeball

3 Which one of the following is NOT a fundamental physical assessment technique?
   a. Percussion
   b. Inspection
   c. Auscultation
   d. Survey
   e. Palpation

4 Which one of the following apertures is used to assess undilated pupils?
   a. Wide angle
   b. Intermediate
   c. Red free
   d. Slit
   e. Fixation target

5 Nails and nail beds are evaluated for which of the following?
   a. Clubbing
   b. Cyanosis

c. Trauma
d. All of the above
e. None of the above

6 The breath of a patient with severe liver disease may smell like which of the following?
   a. Fruity
   b. Urinous
   c. Alcoholic
   d. Sweet
   e. Musty

7 On the anterior view, where is the apex of the lung located?
   a. 3 to 4 cm above the medial end of the clavicles
   b. Between the sixth and eighth ribs
   c. Even with the clavicles
   d. Below the tenth thoracic vertebra
   e. 3 to 4 cm below the medial end of the clavicles

8 A 4+ peripheral pulse is which of the following?
   a. Absent
   b. Moderately impaired
   c. Normal
   d. Markedly impaired
   e. Slightly impaired

9 The normal liver span along the midclavicular line is how long?
   a. 5 cm
   b. 7 cm
   c. 10 cm
   d. 14 cm
   e. 20 cm

10 Interpretation of common proverbs assesses which of the following?
   a. Long-term memory
   b. Abstract thinking
   c. Judgment
   d. Praxis
   e. Affect

CHAPTER 5

Review of Laboratory and Diagnostic Tests

LEARNING OBJECTIVES

1   Differentiate between invasive and noninvasive tests.
2   State the clinical application of common general diagnostic procedures.
3   Identify the clinical application of specific laboratory tests.
4   Identify the clinical application of specific diagnostic procedures.
5   Assess common laboratory and diagnostic test results.

DATA from laboratory and diagnostic tests and procedures provide important information regarding the response to drug therapy, ability of patients to metabolize and eliminate specific therapeutic agents, diagnosis of specific disease, and progression and regression of disease.

This chapter reviews the laboratory and diagnostic tests commonly encountered in the clinical environment. The tests are presented using an organ system approach (i.e., cardiovascular, endocrine, gastrointestinal, hematologic, immunologic, neurologic, renal, respiratory); separate sections on the assessment of infectious diseases and nutritional status also are included. More detailed information about these and other laboratory and diagnostic tests is available in laboratory and medicine textbooks and the current literature.

BACKGROUND |

Laboratory and diagnostic tests are considered either invasive or noninvasive. Invasive tests such as collection of blood (venipuncture) for determining a drug serum concentration and insertion of a central venous catheter for measuring cardiac output and pulmonary artery occlusion pressure involve penetration of the skin or use of instruments that pose some risk to the patient. The degree of risk varies from relatively minor risks such as pain, bleeding, and bruising (associated with venipuncture) to death (associated with more invasive procedures such as coronary angiography). Noninvasive tests such as the taking of chest x-ray films and collection of spontaneously voided urine are associated with minimal risk.

The selection of specific tests and procedures depends on the patient's underlying condition and the need for the information. For example, venipuncture may be considered too invasive and therefore unnecessary for patients with chronic, stable disease but an essential risk when initiating drug treatment in a patient with unstable disease.

Normal laboratory reference values are listed in Tables 5-1 through 5-7.[1-3] However, normal ranges may vary depending on the population and laboratory methodology. Therefore individual patient test results must be interpreted using laboratory-specific reference values. Normal reference values may be reported using conventional units or the Système International d'Unités (SI), which is based on the metric system. Efforts are underway to adopt uniform, internationally accepted systems for the reporting of test results.

GENERAL ORGAN SYSTEM MONITORING

Numerous procedures are available for the diagnosis and monitoring of conditions affecting the various organ systems. The applications and uses of these procedures continue to expand with experience and the integration of new technology.

Laboratory Tests and Diagnostic Procedures

Angiography. Angiography is a radiographic test used to evaluate blood vessels and the circulation. Radiopaque material is injected through a catheter and images are recorded using standard radiographic techniques.

Biopsy. A biopsy involves the removal and evaluation of tissue.

Computed Tomography. Computed tomography (CT) is a technique that uses a computerized x-ray system to produce detailed sectional x-ray images. The system is very sensitive to differences in tissue density and produces detailed, two-dimensional planar images. The tissue attenuation can be increased with the use of contrast agents.

Doppler Echography. Doppler echography uses ultrasound technology to measure shifts in frequency from moving images. For example, Doppler echography is used to evaluate blood flow velocity and turbulence in the heart (Doppler echocardiography) and peripheral circulation.

Fluoroscopy. Fluoroscopy uses a fluoroscope, a device that makes the shadows of x-ray films visible, to provide real-time visualization of procedures. Fluoroscopy exposes a patient to more radiation than does routine radiography but is nevertheless frequently used to visualize needle biopsy and nasogastric tube advancement procedures.

Magnetic Resonance Imaging. Magnetic resonance imaging (MRI) uses an externally applied magnetic field to align the axis of nuclear spin of cellular nuclei. Brief radiofrequency pulses are applied to displace the alignment. Energy emitted when the displacement ends is detected and analyzed to produce finely detailed planar and three-dimensional images. The attenuation can be increased with the use of MRI contrast agents.

Paracentesis. Paracentesis is the removal and analysis of fluid from a body cavity using a hollow instrument.

Plethysmography. Plethysmography measures changes in the size of vessels and hollow organs by measuring displacement of air or fluid from a containing system. For example, body plethysomography is used to assess pulmonary function.

Positron Emission Tomography. Positron emission tomography (PET) imaging uses positron-emitting radionuclides to visualize organs and tissues of the body. The radionuclides decay, producing positrons that collide with electrons. Photons, released when the positrons and electrons collide, are detected by a special camera. This technology can provide quantitative information regarding the structure and function of organs and tissues.

Radionuclide Studies. Radionuclide studies involve the administration (oral, parenteral, inhaled) of radioactive chemicals or pharmaceuticals. X-ray films, usually serial, are taken to record the collection and dispersion of the radioactive material.

Single-Photon Emission Computed Tomography. Single-photon emission computed tomography (SPECT) is similar to PET, but instead involves the administration of radionuclides that emit gamma rays. SPECT is less expensive than PET but provides more limited spatial image resolution.

Standard Radiography (Plain Films, X-Ray Films). Standard radiography produces images on photographic plates by passing roentgen rays through the body. These films are sometimes difficult to interpret because the three dimensionality is lost on planar images.

Ultrasonography (Echography). Ultrasonography uses ultrasound (high-frequency sound waves imperceptible to the human ear) to create images of organs and vessels.

THE CARDIOVASCULAR SYSTEM

A variety of noninvasive and invasive laboratory and diagnostic tests are used to evaluate and monitor the cardiovascular system. The cardiovascular normal reference values are listed in Table 5-1.

Laboratory Tests

Cardiac Enzymes. The pattern and time course of the appearance of enzymes in the blood after cardiac muscle cell damage are used to diagnose myocardial infarction.[4]

Creatine kinase. Creatine kinase (CK) is found in skeletal muscle, cardiac muscle, and the brain, bladder, stomach, and colon. Isoenzyme fractions are used to identify the type of tissue damage. CK-MB is found in cardiac tissue, CK-MM in

Table 5-1	*Adult Cardiovascular Laboratory Reference Values (Based on Serum Tests)*	
INDEX	CONVENTIONAL UNITS	SYSTÈME INTERNATIONAL D'UNITÉS
Creatine kinase		
Female	40-150 U/L	0.67-2.5 μkat/L
Male	60-400 U/L	1-6.67 μkat/L
CK-MB	0-7.5 ng/ml	0-7.5 μg/L
Lactic dehydrogenase	110-210 U/L	1.83-3.50 μkat/L
Lactic dehydrogenase isoenzymes		
LDH_1	17%-27%	0.17-0.27
LDH_2	28%-38%	0.28-0.38
LDH_3	18%-28%	0.18-0.28
LDH_4	5%-15%	0.05-0.15
LDH_5	5%-15%	0.05-0.15
Lipids		
Cholesterol	<200 mg/dl	<5.18 mmol/L
Triglycerides (fasting)	40-150 mg/dl	0.45-1.69 mmol/L

From Jordan CD et al: Normal reference laboratory values, *N Engl J Med* 327:718-724, 1992; Sacher RA, McPherson RA: *Widmann's clinical interpretation of laboratory tests,* ed 10, Philadelphia, 1991, F.A. Davis; Tilkian SM, Conover MB, Tilkian AG: *Clinical implications of laboratory tests,* ed 4, St Louis, 1987, Mosby.

skeletal muscle, and CK-BB in the brain, bladder, stomach, and colon. CK-MB, the gold standard for the diagnosis of acute myocardial infarction, can be detected in the blood within 3 to 5 hours after myocardial infarction; levels peak in about 10 to 20 hours and normalize within about 3 days.

Lactic dehydrogenase. Lactic dehydrogenase (LDH) is found in a variety of body tissues. Isoenzyme fractions are used to identify the type of tissue damage. LDH_1 and LDH_2 are found in the heart, brain, and erythrocytes. LDH_3 is found in the brain and kidney. LDH_4 is found in the liver, skeletal muscle, and kidney. LDH_5 is found in the liver, skeletal muscle, and ileum. LDH_2 normally accounts for the highest percent of total serum LDH. After myocardial infarction the rise in LDH_1 concentration exceeds the rise in LDH_2 concentration (the LDH_1/LDH_2 ratio is greater than 1; a "flipped" ratio). LDH increases within about 12 hours after myocardial infarction, peaks between 24 and 48 hours, and normalizes by about day 10.

Cholesterol. Cholesterol is separated into lipoproteins by protein electrophoresis. Low-density lipoprotein (LDL) is strongly correlated with coronary artery disease. High-density lipoprotein (HDL) is inversely correlated with coronary artery disease.

Lipids. Serum lipids are analyzed as part of the screening process for hyperlipidemias and risk assessment for coronary artery disease. The normal ranges are age and gender dependent.

Myoglobin. Myoglobin is a small protein found in cardiac and skeletal muscle. The presence of myoglobin in the urine or plasma is a relatively sensitive indicator of cellular damage.

Triglycerides. Triglycerides are found in very low-density lipoproteins (VLDLs) and chylomicrons.

Diagnostic Tests and Procedures

Cardiac Catheterization. Cardiac catheterization is used to evaluate cardiac function.[5] A catheter is passed into the right or left side of the heart. Transducers on the tip of the catheter record pressures in the vessels and chambers of the heart. Ports in the catheter provide access for blood samples for the determination of oxygen content and cardiac output.[6] Right-sided catheterization allows for the determination of the right atrial pressures, right ventricular pressures, pulmonary artery pressures, and pulmonary artery occlusion pressure. Left-sided catheterization allows for the determination of left ventricular pressures.

Central Line Placement with Hemodynamic Monitoring. A catheter is placed into the central venous system and advanced into the right side of the heart. The right atrial, right ventricular, pulmonary artery, and pulmonary artery occlusion (formerly known as the pulmonary capillary wedge) pressures can be obtained and cardiac output calculated. These parameters are used to monitor the hemodynamic status of the patient and calculate the pulmonary and peripheral vascular resistances.

Chest Radiography. Chest x-ray films are used to diagnose cardiac disease and monitor the patient's response to drug and nondrug therapy. The size and shape of the atria and ventricles, cardiothoracic ratio, and presence of abnormalities in the lung fields and pleural spaces can be determined by assessment of chest x-ray films.

Coronary Angiography. The cardiac vessels are visualized by injecting a contrast agent through the catheter tip.

Digital Subtraction Angiography. In digital subtraction angiography (DSA), background images are obtained before the contrast agent is injected and then "subtracted" from the images obtained after the injection of the contrast agent. This technique improves the resolution of the image.

Echocardiography. Echocardiography is used to evaluate the size, shape, and motion of the valves, septum, and walls and changes in chamber size during the cardiac cycle.[7] The beam may be applied to the heart through the chest (transthoracic approach) or esophagus (transesophageal approach).

Contrast echocardiography. Visualization of the right-sided chambers of the heart is enhanced by the injection of contrast agents.

Doppler echocardiography. Doppler and echocardiography techniques may be combined to evaluate cardiac blood flow patterns.

Exercise echocardiography. Exercise echocardiography compares echocardiograms obtained before and during exercise.

M-mode echocardiography. M-mode echocardiography records the motion of the heart over time. It is used to evaluate the structures of the heart throughout the cardiac cycle.

Two-dimensional echocardiography. Two-dimensional echocardiography records a two-dimensional image of the heart. The spatial anatomic relationships can be determined by changing the angle of the beam.

Electrocardiography. Electrocardiography is the recording and assessment of electrocardiograms.

Electrocardiogram. The electrocardiogram (ECG) provides a record of the electrical activity of the heart at rest.[8] It is used to diagnose cardiac disease, monitor the response to drug therapy, and monitor for adverse drug effects.

Electrocardiogram with stress (stress test). The ECG is recorded during a standardized exercise protocol with gradually increasing levels of exercise[9,10] or with the patient at rest after the administration of dobutamine or dipyridamole; either intervention increases myocardial oxygen consumption and blood flow. A motorized treadmill or cycle ergometer is used for the exercise stress test. Blood pressure, heart rate, oxygen consumption, oxygen saturation, and arterial blood gas data are commonly collected to provide a thorough assessment of the function of the cardiovascular system under stress conditions.

Holter monitoring (ambulatory electrocardiography). The ECG is recorded continuously using a portable recorder. This method provides prolonged monitoring with unrestricted activity.

Thallium stress test. The thallium stress test combines the parenteral administration of thallium-201, a radionuclide taken up by healthy myocardial tissue and the stress test (either exercise or pharmacologic). A gamma camera is used to record serial images of the myocardium.

Intracardiac Electrophysiologic Studies. Intracardiac electrophysiologic studies (EPSs) are tests in which special catheters with electrodes are used to stimulate the cardiac tissue to assess the nature and origin of cardiac arrhythmias and the response to antiarrhythmic drug therapy.

Lymphoscintigraphy. Lymphoscintigraphy evaluates the patency and anatomy of peripheral lymph vessels by depositing a radioactive agent in the tissue drained by the lymph system being evaluated.[11,12] The test is used to assess lymphedema and tumor involvement of regional lymph nodes inaccessible to other imaging procedures.

Multiple Gated Acquisition Scan. The multiple gated acquisition (MUGA) scan, also known as *radionuclide angiocardiography,* evaluates ventricular function, cardiac wall motion, ejection fraction, and cardiac output after the injection of radionuclide-labeled (technetium 99m) albumin or red blood cells.[13]

Technetium 99m Pyrophosphate Uptake. Infarcted myocardial tissue has an increased uptake of technetium 99m compared with normal tissue. The isotope is injected parenterally and serial images of the heart are obtained to evaluate the location and extent of the myocardial infarction.

THE ENDOCRINE SYSTEM

The endocrine system consists of the pituitary, hypothalamus, adrenal gland, thyroid gland, parathyroid glands, and pancreas. The endocrine system is assessed by measuring the levels of the hormones produced by the different components of the system.[14,15] Therapeutic response to replacement or suppressive drug therapy also is assessed by measuring the levels of these hormones. A variety of specific tests are used to assess each component of the endocrine system. The normal endocrine reference values are listed in Table 5-2.

Laboratory Tests
Adrenal Tests
Adrenal medulla. The adrenal medulla secretes catecholamines. The 24-hour urinary excretion of epinephrine, norepinephrine, and vanillylmandelic acid (VMA) is used to assess the function of the adrenal medulla.

Adrenal cortex. The adrenal cortex secretes mineralocorticoids, glucocorticoids, and androgens. Tests used to assess the function of the adrenal cortex include plasma and urine aldosterone, plasma renin activity, serum testosterone, serum estradiol, plasma cortisol (morning and evening), plasma adrenocorticotropic hormone (ACTH) (morning), and urinary excretion rates of the 17-hydroxycorticosteroids, 17-ketogenic steroids, and 17-ketosteroids.

Dexamethasone Suppression Test. A baseline 8 a.m. plasma cortisol level is obtained and then 1 mg of dexamethasone is administered orally at 11 p.m. Normally cortisol production is suppressed, and the 8 a.m. plasma cortisol level obtained the next day is low.

Human Chorionic Gonadotropin. Human chorionic gonadotropin (HCG) is produced by the placenta. It is detected in the urine as early as 10 days after a missed menstrual cycle and peaks at about 10 weeks.

Insulin Tolerance Test. Insulin (0.05 to 0.1 U/kg) is administered intravenously. Serial blood samples are obtained for 90 minutes. ACTH is released when the blood glucose falls to less than 40 mg/dl.

Metyrapone Test. Metyrapone inhibits the final step in cortisol synthesis. For this test, 500 to 750 mg of metyrapone is administered orally every 4 hours for 24 hours and plasma samples are collected. A normal response is a decrease in plasma cortisol and an elevation in urine and plasma 11-deoxycortisol (compound S).

Pancreatic Tests
Amylase. Amylase is secreted by the pancreas, bowel, parotids, and gynecologic system. Although not specific for pancreatitis, serum amylase is easier to measure than is lipase and is used as a common screening and monitoring parameter for acute pancreatitis. However, in chronic pancreatitis the pancreas may be "burned out" and unable to secrete amylase.

C peptide. C peptide is an inactive peptide chain released from beta cells in equimolar amounts with insulin and found in the serum in about a 5:1 to 15:1 ratio with insulin. C peptide is sometimes used to assess pancreatic function.

		CONVENTIONAL	SYSTÈME INTERNATIONAL
Table 5-2 *Adult Endocrine Laboratory Reference Values*			
INDEX	SOURCE	UNITS	D'UNITÉS
THYROID			
Free thyroxine index		4.6-11.2	4.6-11.2
Thyroid-stimulating hormone	S*	0.5-5 μU/ml	0.5-5mU/L
Total triiodothyronine (T$_3$)	S	75-195 ng/dl	1.2-3.0 nmol/L
Total thyroxine (T$_4$)	S	4-12 μg/dl	51-154 nmol/L
PITUITARY			
Adrenocorticotropic hormone (ACTH)	P†	6-76 pg/ml	1.3-16.7 pmol/L
Growth hormone (fasting)	P	2-6 ng/ml	2-6 μg/L
Prolactin			
Female	S	0-15 ng/ml	0-15 μg/L
Male	S	0-10 ng/ml	0-10 μg/L
ADRENAL CORTEX			
Aldosterone (recumbent, normal salt diet)	S,P	<16 ng/dl	<444 pmol/L
Cortisol (8 a.m. fasting)	P	0-10 μg/dl	0-276 nmol/L
Renin (supine) (6 hr, recumbent, normal salt diet)	P	0.5-1.6 ng/ml/hr	0.14-0.44 ng/(L × sec)
ADRENAL MEDULLA AND CATECHOL SECRETIONS			
Epinephrine	U‡	1.7-22.4 μg/day	9.3-122 nmol/day
Norepinephrine	U	12.1-85.5 μg/day	72-505 nmol/day
Vanillylmandelic acid (VMA)	U	1.4-6.5 mg/day	7.1-32.7 μmol/day
GONADAL HORMONES			
Estradiol			
Female			
Premenopausal	S,P	23-361 pg/ml	84-1325 pmol/L
Postmenopausal	S,P	<30 pg/ml	<110 pmol/L
Male	S,P	<50 pg/ml	<184 pmol/L
Testosterone			
Female	P	20-90 ng/dl	0.7-3.1 nmol/L
Male	P	300-1100 ng/dl	10.4-38.1 nmol/L
PANCREATIC			
Amylase	S	53-123 U/L	0.88-2.05 nkat/L
Glucose (fasting)	P	70-110 mg/dl	3.9-5.6 mmol/L
Insulin (fasting)	S	0-29 μU/ml	0-208 pmol/L
Lipase	S	4-24 U/dl	0.67-4 μkat/L
PARATHYROID			
Calcium	S	8.5-10.5 mg/dl	2.1-2.6 mmol/L
Parathyroid hormone	P	10-60 pg/ml	10-60 ng/L
Phosphorus	S	2.6-4.5 mg/dl	0.84-1.45 mmol/L

From Jordan CD et al: Normal reference laboratory values, *N Engl J Med* 327:718-724, 1992; Sacher RA, McPherson RA: *Widmann's clinical interpretation of laboratory tests*, ed 10, Philadelphia, 1991, F.A. Davis; Tilkian SM, Conover MB, Tilkian AG: *Clinical implications of laboratory tests*, ed 4, St Louis, 1987, Mosby.
*S, Serum.
†P, Plasma.
‡U, Urine.

Glucose. Serum glucose concentrations are used to assess pancreatic function and the response to insulin replacement therapy.

Fasting serum glucose. The serum sample is obtained after 10 to 14 hours of fasting. The fasting serum glucose is usually obtained before breakfast after an overnight fast.

Glucose tolerance test. The glucose tolerance test (GTT) is used to diagnose diabetes mellitus and gestational diabetes. Patients fast for 10 to 16 hours before the test and are then given approximately 75 g of glucose. Serial blood samples are obtained and the serum glucose concentration is determined. Normally the serum blood glucose is less than 200 mg/dl at 30, 60, and 90 minutes and less than 140 mg/dl at 2 hours.

Random serum glucose. The random serum glucose sample can be obtained at any time without fasting.

Glycosylated hemoglobin. Glycosylated hemoglobin is formed when hemoglobin is irreversibly glycosylated after exposure to high glucose levels. Glycosylated hemoglobin is sometimes used to assess long-term control of insulin therapy and differentiate factitious hyperglycemia from diabetes.

Insulin. Fasting serum insulin is sometimes obtained during the assessment of pancreatic function.

Lipase. Lipase is a specific marker for acute pancreatic disease. Increases in serum lipase parallel increases in serum amylase. However, in chronic pancreatitis the pancreas may be "burned out" and unable to secrete lipase.

Parathyroid Tests. The parathyroid gland secretes parathyroid hormone (PTH). High serum calcium levels suppress PTH secretion. Parathyroid gland function is tested by measuring the serum concentrations of parathyroid hormone, calcium, and phosphorus. The serum concentration of PTH is useful in differentiating between hypercalcemia resulting from hyperparathyroidism and hypercalcemia resulting from other causes.

Pituitary Tests

Anterior pituitary. The anterior pituitary hormones include growth hormone, prolactin, thyroid stimulating hormone, follicle-stimulating hormone, luteinizing hormone, and adrenocorticotropic hormone (ACTH). Pituitary function is assessed by measuring the concentrations of the hormones at baseline and after stimulation or suppression tests.

Adrenocorticotropic hormone stimulation test. For the ACTH stimulation test a baseline plasma cortisol level is obtained and then 250 mcg of cosyntropin is injected intravenously. Normally, plasma cortisol levels peak in 30 to 60 minutes.

Posterior pituitary. The posterior pituitary hormones include antidiuretic hormone and oxytocin. Tests used to evaluate posterior pituitary function include concentration testing and water loading. Concentration testing involves overnight water deprivation and evaluation of urine and serum osmolality. Water loading involves administering 1000 ml of water and then evaluating urine and serum osmolality.

Thyroid Tests. Thyroid function tests are used to establish the level of thyroid function (e.g., hyperthyroid, hypothyroid, euthyroid) and response to suppressant or replacement therapy. Thyroid function is assessed by evaluating the serum concentrations of the free hormones thyroxine (T_4) and triiodothyronine (T_3) and by a number of indirect methods.

Free thyroxine index. The free thyroxine index (FT_4I) is the product of the measured T_4 and the triiodothyronine uptake (T_3U). It takes into account the absolute hormone level and the binding capacity of thyroid-binding globulin. The FT_4I is decreased in hypothyroidism and increased in hyperthyroidism.

Thyroid-stimulating hormone (thyrotropin). Serum thyroid-stimulating hormone (TSH), or thyrotropin, levels are used to differentiate between thyroid hypothyroidism and pituitary hypothyroidism. The TSH level is elevated in thyroidal hypothyroidism and markedly decreased in pituitary hypothyroidism.

Thyroid uptake of radioiodine. Radioactive iodine (^{123}I or ^{131}I) is administered orally and the radioactivity over the thyroid gland is counted at various intervals. The normal radioactive iodine uptake (RAIU) is about 10% to 35%.

Thyrotropin-releasing hormone. Thyrotropin-releasing hormone (TRH) stimulates the pituitary to release TSH. Injection of synthetic TRH normally causes an increase in TSH in about 30 minutes.

Triiodothyronine uptake. The triiodothyronine uptake (T_3U) test is an in vitro test that indirectly estimates the amount of thyroid-binding globulin in the serum.

THE GASTROINTESTINAL SYSTEM

A variety of noninvasive and invasive laboratory and diagnostic tests are used to evaluate and monitor the gastrointestinal system. The normal gastrointestinal reference values are listed in Table 5-3.

Laboratory Tests

Biliary System. Bilirubin is useful in the diagnosis and monitoring of liver disease and hemolytic anemia and the assessment of the severity of jaundice. A patient is generally visibly jaundiced if the bilirubin level is greater than 2 mg/dl.

Alkaline phosphatase. Alkaline phosphatase is elevated in biliary cirrhosis, cirrhosis, and intrahepatic bile duct disease.

Direct bilirubin. Direct bilirubin is the conjugated posthepatic bilirubin. It is increased in obstructive jaundice.

Indirect bilirubin. Indirect bilirubin is the unconjugated bilirubin. It is increased in hemolytic jaundice and liver cell damage.

Total bilirubin. Total bilirubin is the combination of direct and indirect bilirubin.

Hepatocellular Function

Synthetic function. Many drugs are hepatically metabolized. One way of assessing the ability of the liver to metabolize these agents is to assess the synthetic function of the liver by evaluating the quantity of specific products produced or processed by it.[16] These include ammonia, albumin, and the vitamin K–dependent clotting factors.

Ammonia. The liver synthesizes urea from ammonia. Serum ammonia is increased if the liver is damaged or blood flow is compromised. Although the serum ammonia is not used as a screening test, it is sometimes used to confirm a diagnosis of hepatic encephalopathy.

Protein production. The liver manufactures many different proteins. The serum albumin and the vitamin K–dependent clotting factors are commonly used to assess hepatic synthetic function.

ALBUMIN. Although circulating albumin takes several weeks to clear from the body, a rapidly declining serum protein level indicates greatly impaired hepatic function. Long-standing liver disease is associated with very low serum protein concentrations.

Table 5-3	*Adult Gastrointestinal Laboratory Reference Values*		
INDEX	SOURCE	CONVENTIONAL UNITS	SYSTÈME INTERNATIONAL D'UNITÉS
Alanine aminotransferase (ALT)			
Female	S*	7-30 U/L	0.12-0.50 μkat/L
Male	S	10-55 U/L	0.17-0.91 μkat/L
Alkaline phosphatase			
Female	S	30-100 U/L	0.5-1.67 μkat/L
Male	S	45-115 U/L	0.75-1.92 μkat/L
Ammonia	P†	12-55 μmol/L	12-55 μmol/L
Aspartate aminotransferase (AST)			
Female	S	9-25 U/L	0.15-0.42 μkat/L
Male	S	10-40 U/L	0.17-0.67 μkat/L
Bilirubin			
Direct	S	Up to 0.4 mg/dl	Up to 7 μmol/L
Total	S	Up to 1 mg/dl	Up to 17 μmol/L
Gamma-glutamyl transpeptidase (GGT)	S	1-60 U/L	0.02-1 μkat/L
Lactic dehydrogenase (LDH)	S	110-210 U/L	1.83-3.5 μkat/L
Partial thromboplastin time, activated (aPTT)	P	24-37 sec	24-37 sec
Protein			
Albumin	S	3.1-4.3 g/dl	31-43 g/L
Globulin	S	2.6-4.1 g/dl	26-31 g/L
Total	S	6-8 g/dl	60-80 g/L
Prothrombin time (PT)	P	8.8-11.6 sec	8.8-11.6 sec
Stool fat	Stool	1-7 g/day	3.5-25 mmol/day

From Jordan CD et al: Normal reference laboratory values, *N Engl J Med* 327:718-724, 1992; Sacher RA, McPherson RA: *Widmann's clinical interpretation of laboratory tests,* ed 10, Philadelphia, 1991, F.A. Davis; Tilkian SM, Conover MB, Tilkian AG: *Clinical implications of laboratory tests,* ed 4, St Louis, 1987, Mosby.
*S, Serum.
†P, Plasma.

VITAMIN K–DEPENDENT CLOTTING FACTORS (FACTORS II, VII, IX, AND X). Lack of production of the vitamin K–dependent clotting factors prolongs the prothrombin time (PT) and partial thromboplastin time (PTT). The PT is prolonged earlier than the PTT and is often used as an early indicator of impaired hepatic synthetic function. Both the PT and PTT are prolonged in long-standing severe hepatic dysfunction.

Transaminases. The serum transaminases are increased if cells are damaged and enzymes released into the circulation.[17] Elevations occur in the presence of marked changes in circulation (such as shock) and diseases associated with hepatocellular damage (hepatitis, cirrhosis, inflammatory diseases, and infiltrative hepatic diseases). The serum enzymes may not be markedly elevated in severe, chronic, end-stage liver disease ("burned out" liver). Very high elevations (more than 20 times normal) are associated with viral or toxic hepatitis. Moderately high elevations (3 to 10 times normal) are associated with infectious mononucleosis, chronic active hepatitis, extrahepatic bile duct obstruction, and intrahepatic cholestasis. Modest elevations (one to three times normal) are associated with pancreatitis, alcoholic fatty liver, biliary cirrhosis, and neoplastic infiltration.

Alanine aminotransferase. Alanine aminotransferase (ALT) is found in high concentrations in hepatocytes and is considered a specific marker of hepatocellular damage.

Aspartate aminotransferase. Aspartate aminotransferase (AST) is found in hepatocytes, myocardial muscles, skeletal muscle, and the brain and kidney. It is used as a nonspecific marker of hepatocellular damage.

Gamma glutamyl transpeptidase. Gamma glutamyl transpeptidase (GGT) is found in hepatobiliary, pancreatic, and kidney cells. It is elevated in most hepatocellular and hepatobiliary disease, although elevations correlate better with obstructive disease than with pure hepatocellular damage. An elevated GGT level is often one of the early indicators of alcoholic liver disease.

Lactic dehydrogenase. Lactic dehydrogenase (LDH) is found in the heart, brain, erythrocytes, kidney, liver, skeletal muscle, and ileum. Elevations occur during shock syndrome (marked changes in circulation) and diseases associated with hepatocellular damage (hepatitis, cirrhosis, inflammatory disease, and infiltrative diseases).

Stool. The stool is evaluated for color, consistency, and the presence of obvious or occult blood, fat, ova and parasites, microorganisms, and white blood cells. The color of the stool provides important diagnostic and monitoring information. Black stools are generally associated with upper gastrointestinal tract bleeding; however, iron therapy may produce a similar color. Red stools are generally associated with lower gastrointestinal tract bleeding. Gray stools are generally associated with steatorrhea. Light gray stools are generally associated with bile duct obstruction. Watery stools are indicative of rapid gastrointestinal transit and malabsorption syndromes. Hard stools may indicate dehydration. The presence of obvious blood in the stool is generally associated with colonic bleeding. Occult blood, present with both upper and lower gastrointestinal tract bleeding, may be identified for several weeks after gastrointestinal bleeding. Stool fat is increased in diseases associated with altered bacterial flora, increased gastrointestinal motility, decreased enzyme and bile acid content, and loss of absorptive surfaces. White blood cells are associated with a variety of infectious processes and inflammatory bowel disease.

Miscellaneous

Alpha-fetoprotein. Alpha-fetoprotein is the major protein produced by the fetus in the first 10 weeks of life. It also is produced by rapidly multiplying hepatocytes and is used as a marker of hepatocellular carcinoma.

Carcinoembryonic antigen. The carcinoembryonic antigen (CEA) is a tumor marker found in the blood. It is associated with rapid multiplication of digestive system epithelial cells and is used to monitor tumor recurrence.

Diagnostic Tests and Procedures

Abdominal Radiography. The abdominal x-ray film, including the kidneys, ureter, and bladder (KUB), is taken with the patient supine on the back.

Barium Studies. Contrast material such as barium sulfate is swallowed and x-ray films are taken to visualize the esophagus, stomach, and small intestine. Barium enemas are used to visualize the large intestine. The double-contrast barium enema technique uses the combination of barium and air to visualize the large intestine and is considered a more precise procedure.

Cholecystosonography. Sonography is used to detect gallstones and evaluate the gallbladder, biliary system, and adjacent organs. Sonography has nearly replaced cholecystography.

Cholescystography. Cholecystography is used to evaluate gallbladder function and anatomy. Orally administered iopanoic acid concentrates in the gallbladder, opacifying it.[18]

Colonoscopy. A flexible fiberoptic tube is inserted rectally to visualize the lining of the large intestine.

d-Xylose Test. The d-xylose test is used to screen for carbohydrate malabsorption.[19] For this test a dose of 25 g of d-xylose is administered with water, and the urine is collected for a 5-hour period. Normally more than 3 g of d-xylose is excreted in the urine during this period.

Endoscopic Retrograde Cholangiopancreatography. In endoscopic retrograde cholangiopancreatography (ERCP) the biliary system and pancreatic duct are visualized by inserting a catheter into the ampulla of Vater and injecting contrast material into the biliary system.

Endoscopy. A flexible fiberoptic tube is inserted orally to visualize the lining of the esophagus, stomach, duodenum, ampulla of Vater, and biliary and pancreatic systems.

Intragastric pH. The pH of gastric secretions is sometimes measured to monitor the effectiveness of antacid or H_2-receptor antagonist drug therapy.

Manometry. Manometry is used to evaluate esophageal contractions and esophageal sphincter pressures.[20] Pressures are measured by pressure transducers on a tube inserted orally.

Percutaneous Transhepatic Cholangiogram. Contrast media is injected directly into the biliary radicle within the liver and fluoroscopy is used to visualize the intrahepatic and extrahepatic bile ducts.

pH Stimulation Tests. Tests involving pH stimulation are used to determine the response of gastric acid secretion to a chemical stimulus; they are sometimes used to diagnose hyposecretory and hypersecretory gastric acid disorders. Gastric secretions are collected from the stomach by aspiration through a nasogastric tube. Secretions are collected at baseline and after stimulation with betazole or pentagastrin.

Schilling Test. The Schilling test is used to evaluate the absorption of vitamin B_{12} (cyanocobalamin). In the first part of the test, 1000 mcg of regular B_{12} is administered parenterally to saturate the systemic vitamin B_{12} storage sites. A 0.5 to 1 mcg dose of ^{57}Co-labeled vitamin B_{12} is then administered orally and urine is collected. Normally more than 7% of the radiolabeled vitamin B_{12} is excreted in the urine in a 24-hour period. If indicated the test may be repeated with the administration of 60 mcg of oral intrinsic factor. If the malabsorption of vitamin B_{12} is caused by a deficiency of intrinsic factor, the amount of radiolabeled B_{12} excreted in the urine rises to normal levels.

Sigmoidoscopy. An endoscope is used to evaluate the gastrointestinal tract from the anus to about 60 cm of the terminal colon. The rigid sigmoidoscope is used to screen for rectosigmoid cancer, obtain large mucosal biopsies, and evaluate patients with inflammatory disease of the rectum or distal sigmoid colon. The flexible sigmoidoscope is longer and more useful in the assessment of the sigmoid colon.

THE HEMATOLOGIC SYSTEM |

Blood consists of plasma and blood cells suspended in the plasma. The plasma consists of water and dissolved proteins, electrolytes, and organic and inorganic substances. The blood cells consist of erythrocytes, or red blood cells (RBCs); leukocytes, or white blood cells (WBCs); and platelets. A variety of noninvasive and invasive laboratory and diagnostic tests are used to evaluate and monitor the hematologic system. The normal hematology reference values are listed in Table 5-4.

General Laboratory Tests

ABO Blood Typing. The antigenic properties of blood are typed to avoid potentially lethal transfusion reactions. Blood types include A, B, AB, and O.

Blood Smear. The blood smear is produced by smearing a drop of peripheral blood on a slide and examining the smear microscopically. The blood smear is used to obtain a WBC count and differential, estimate the platelet count, and evaluate RBC morphology.

Coagulation Tests. The common tests of coagulation include the bleeding time, partial thromboplastin time, prothrombin time, and thrombin time.

Bleeding time. The bleeding time is the duration of bleeding after a standardized skin incision. It is used to evaluate platelet quantity and function.

Partial thromboplastin time. The partial thromboplastin time (PTT) assesses the intrinsic clotting pathway. It is commonly used to monitor heparin therapy.

Prothrombin time. The prothrombin time (PT) assesses the extrinsic clotting pathway. It is used to monitor warfarin therapy and assess hepatic synthetic function. The international normalized ratio (INR) is a more standardized expression of prothrombin time that takes into account differences in reagent activity. It is calculated according to the equation $INR = (PT_{patient} \div PT_{control})^{ISI}$, where ISI is the International Sensitivity Index.

Thrombin time. The thrombin time is used to evaluate the effect of heparin and thrombolytic drug therapy and coagulation abnormalities.

Complete Blood Count. The complete blood count (CBC) consists of the hemoglobin, hematocrit, RBC count, WBC count, mean corpuscular volume, mean corpuscular hemoglobin, and mean corpuscular hemoglobin concentration.

Crossmatching. Crossmatching determines compatibility between the donor's and patient's blood. Agglutination between the donor's red cells and the recipient's serum indicates incompatibility.

Fibrinogen. Fibrinogen is increased in disseminated intravascular coagulation. It is used to evaluate bleeding disorders.

Fibrin Degradation Products. Fibrin degradation products (FDPs) are released when fibrin is broken down. They are assessed in the diagnosis and monitoring of disseminated intravascular coagulation.

Hemoglobin Electrophoresis. Immunoelectrophoresis uses electrophoretic separation and immunodiffusion to screen for the presence of abnormal proteins such as Bence Jones and myeloma proteins.

Serum Protein Electrophoresis. Serum protein electrophoresis (SPEP) is used to screen for serum protein abnormalities. The proteins (albumin, α-1 globulin, α-2 globulin, beta globulin, and gamma globulin) are identified by different migration patterns they follow when subjected to an electric field.

			SYSTÈME INTERNATIONAL
INDEX	SOURCE	CONVENTIONAL	D'UNITÉS

Table 5-4 *Adult Hematology Reference Laboratory Values*

INDEX	SOURCE	CONVENTIONAL	SYSTÈME INTERNATIONAL D'UNITÉS
Bleeding time		2-9.5 min	2-9.5 min
Blood volume		8.5%-9.5% of body weight in kg	80-85 ml/kg
Erythrocyte count	WB*	$4.15\text{-}4.9 \times 10^6/mm^3$	$4.15\text{-}4.9 \times 10^{12}/L$
Erythrocyte sedimentation rate			
Female	WB	1-30 mm/hr	1-30 mm/hr
Male	WB	1-13 mm/hr	1-13 mm/hr
Ferritin	S†	>20 ng/ml	>20 μg/L
Fibrin degradation products	S	<10 μg/ml	<100 mg/L
Folic acid	S	≥3.3 ng/ml	>7.3 nmol/L
Hematocrit			
Female	WB	37%-48%	0.37-0.48
Male	WB	42%-52%	0.42-0.52
Hemoglobin			
Female	WB	12-16 g/dl	7.4-9.9 mmol/L
Male	WB	13-18 g/dl	8.1-11.2 mmol/L
Iron	S	50-150 μg/dl	9-26.9 μmol/L
Iron-binding capacity	S	250-410 μg/dl	45-73 μmol/L
Leukocyte count	WB	$4.3\text{-}10.8 \times 10^3/mm^3$	$4.3\text{-}10.8 \times 10^9/L$
T lymphocytes	WB	74%-86% of circulating lymphocytes	74%-86% of circulating lymphocytes
B lymphocytes	WB	5%-25% of circulating lymphocytes	5%-25% of circulating lymphocytes
T4 lymphocytes (CD4)	WB	38%-52% of circulating lymphocytes	38%-52% of circulating lymphocytes
T8 lymphocytes (CD8)	WB	22%-36% of circulating lymphocytes	22%-36% of circulating lymphocytes
T4/T8 ratio		1.0:2.2	1.0:2.2
Mean corpuscular volume (MCV)	WB	86-98 μm^3	86-98 fl
Mean corpuscular hemoglobin (MCH)	WB	28-33 pg/cell	28-33 pg/cell
Mean corpuscular hemoglobin concentration (MCHC)	WB	32-36 g/dl	320-360 g/L
Partial thromboplastin time, activated (aPTT)	P‡	24-37 sec	24-37 sec
Platelet count	WB	$150\text{-}350 \times 10^3/mm^3$	$150\text{-}350 \times 10^9/L$
Prothrombin time (PT)	P	8.8-11.6 sec	8.8-11.6 sec
Red cell distribution width	WB	11.5%-14.5%	0.115-0.145
Reticulocyte count	WB	0.5%-2.5% of red cells	0.005-0.025 red cells
Thrombin time	P	Control ± 5 sec	Control ± 5 sec
Vitamin B$_{12}$	S	205-876 pg/ml	151-674 pmol/L

From Jordan CD et al: Normal reference laboratory values, *N Engl J Med* 327:718-724, 1992; Sacher RA, McPherson RA: *Widmann's clinical interpretation of laboratory tests,* ed 10, Philadelphia, 1991, F.A. Davis; Tilkian SM, Conover MB, Tilkian AG: *Clinical implications of laboratory tests,* ed 4, St Louis, 1987, Mosby.
*WB, Whole blood.
†S, Serum.
‡P, Plasma.

Laboratory Tests by Specific Cell Type

Platelets. Platelets are responsible for initiating hemostasis. The risk of spontaneous bleeding is greatly increased if the platelet count is less than 20,000 cells/mm^3. The platelet count is sometimes estimated from the peripheral blood smear; it is considered adequate if the smear contains two to three platelets per field. The count may be performed manually or electronically and is a more accurate estimate of the number of platelets.

The platelet count and function may be altered in a variety of diseases. The platelet count may be decreased if the bone marrow fails to produce platelets (such as in aplastic anemia, leukemia, and some viral infections) or if increased peripheral destruction of platelets occurs (such as in idiopathic thrombocytopenic purpura, some collagen vascular diseases, thrombotic thrombocytopenic purpura, disseminated intravascular coagulation, and hemolytic uremic syndrome). The platelet count may be increased after splenectomy, in some myeloproliferative diseases such as myelogenous leukemia and essential thrombocythemia, and in chronic inflammatory diseases, malignancy, and chronic infections. Platelet function may be impaired by drugs such as aspirin, dipyridamole, and nonsteroidal antiinflammatory drugs and disease states such as uremia, multiple myeloma, and severe liver disease.

Red Blood Cells

Carboxyhemoglobin. Carboxyhemoglobin is formed when carbon monoxide is inhaled. The carbon monoxide attaches to hemoglobin, rendering the hemoglobin incapable of carrying oxygen.

Coombs' test. The Coombs' test is performed using an antiserum containing antibodies that act to bridge antibody- or complement-coated RBCs. Agglutination occurs when the cells are bridged.

Direct Coombs' test. The direct Coombs' test uses antibodies directed against human proteins (primarily immunoglobulin G [IgG] and complement [C3]) to detect whether these proteins are attached to the surface of RBCs. The direct Coombs' test is used to differentiate between immunologic (e.g., autoimmune) and nonimmunologic (e.g., drug-induced) hemolytic anemias.

Indirect Coombs' test. The indirect Coombs' test detects antibodies against human RBCs in the patient's serum. The indirect Coombs' test is used in crossmatching before transfusion.

Erythrocyte sedimentation rate. The erythrocyte sedimentation rate (ESR) is a nonspecific indicator of inflammation. This test measures the rate at which RBCs settle out of mixed venous blood. The rate of settling is influenced by the shape of the RBC and the charges on the membrane. It is used as a nonspecific marker of inflammatory and malignant disease.

Folate. Decreased serum folate levels are associated with megaloblastic anemias.

Hematocrit. The hematocrit is the number of RBCs in 100 ml of blood reported as a percentage. Normal reference values vary with age, gender, and elevation above sea level. The hematocrit is increased in vitamin B_{12} and folic acid deficiencies and decreased in iron deficiency. The hematocrit is used to diagnose anemia and assess response to replacement therapy.

Hemoglobin. Hemoglobin is the oxygen-carrying protein in RBCs. Normal reference values vary with age, gender, and elevation above sea level. Hemoglobin is decreased in blood loss and iron deficiency anemia. Hemoglobin is used to diagnose anemia, assess response to replacement therapy, and estimate oxygen content.

Iron metabolism

Ferritin. Serum ferritin does not contain iron, but is in equilibrium with tissue ferritin, making it a useful indicator of tissue iron stores. It is used to diagnose iron deficiency anemia.

Iron. Serum iron levels are decreased in iron deficiency anemia, chronic infections, and some malignancies. Serum iron levels may be increased in iron poisoning and hemolysis.

Total iron-binding capacity. The total iron-binding capacity (TIBC) test evaluates the capacity of transferrin to bind to iron. It is used to diagnose iron deficiency anemia and monitor replacement therapy.

Transferrin saturation. Transferrin is a specific iron transport protein. This test evaluates the percent of total iron-binding protein saturated with iron. It is used to diagnose iron deficiency anemia and monitor replacement therapy.

Red blood cell appearance. The size, shape, and color of RBCs is influenced by many diseases. A variety of terms are used to describe the RBC appearance:

Acanthocytes. Acanthocytes are RBCs with long, thin, irregularly placed spines on the membrane; they are associated with alcoholic cirrhosis and heparin therapy and may occur after splenectomy.

Anisocytosis. Aniscytosis is the presence of variable RBC size; it is associated with early iron replacement therapy.

Burr cells. Burr cells are RBCs with evenly distributed spicules on the membrane; they are associated with uremia.

Elliptocytes. Elliptocytes are rod-shaped RBCs; they are associated with sickle cell trait and thalassemia.

Hypochromia. Hypochromia is a decrease in the hemoglobin content of the RBCs. It produces pale red blood cells and is associated with folic acid and vitamin B_{12} deficiency anemias.

Macrocytes. Macrocytes are larger than normal RBCs.

Microcytes. Microcytes are smaller than normal RBCs.

Normochromia. The term *normochromia* describes the normal color of the RBCs.

Normocytes. Normocytes are normal-sized RBCs.

Ovalocytes. Ovalocytes are oval-shaped RBCs; they are associated with microcytic and megaloblastic anemias.

Schistocytes. Schistocytes are fragments of RBCs; they are associated with disseminated intravascular coagulation, prosthetic heart valves, uremia, and sickle cell anemia.

Spherocytes. Spherocytes are small, round RBCs; they are associated with anemias and hemolytic transfusion reactions.

Stomatocytes. Stomatocytes are RBCs with central slitlike areas of pallor; they are associated with neoplastic, liver, and cardiac disease.

Target cells. Target cells are RBCs with dark centers surrounded by light rings; they are associated with sickle cell anemia, iron deficiency, and liver disease; they also may occur after splenectomy.

Red blood cell count. The RBC count is the number of RBCs per ml of blood. It is used to diagnose anemias and assess response to replacement therapy. It also serves as an indicator of chronic hypoxemia.

Red blood cell inclusions. RBCs may contain abnormal material, known as *inclusions*.

Basophilic stippling. Basophilic stippling is fine stippling that is associated with lead poisoning and some anemias.

Heinz bodies. Heinz bodies are masses of denatured hemoglobin; they are associated with severe oxidative stress and thalassemia.

Howell-Jolly bodies. Howell-Jolly bodies are fragments of nuclear deoxyribonucleic acid (DNA) that appear as dark purple dots; they may occur after splenectomy and also are associated with hemolytic and megaloblastic anemias.

Nucleated red blood cells. Nucleated RBCs are less mature RBCs with nuclei; they are associated with intense marrow erythropoietic activity.

Red blood cell indices. The RBC indices consist of the mean cell volume, mean cell hemoglobin, and mean cell hemoglobin concentration. These indices are used in the differential diagnosis of anemia and for monitoring response to replacement therapy.

Mean cell hemoglobin. Mean cell hemoglobin (MCH) is the average RBC hemoglobin content. MCH is decreased in iron deficiency anemias and increased in folic acid and vitamin B_{12} deficiencies. It is increased in hemolytic anemias.

Mean cell hemoglobin concentration. Mean cell hemoglobin concentration (MCHC) is the amount of hemoglobin per volume of RBCs.

Mean cell volume. Mean cell volume (MCV) is the average volume of the individual RBCs. MCV is decreased in iron deficiency anemias, thalassemias, and chronic diseases, resulting in microcytic anemias. It is increased in folic acid and vitamin B_{12} deficiencies, resulting in macrocytic anemias.

Red cell distribution width. The red cell distribution width (RDW) is a histogram of the distribution of red cell volumes as measured by automated equipment. It is used to diagnose anemias and assess response to replacement therapy.

Reticulocytes. Reticulocytes are immature RBCs that contain residual ribonucleic acid (RNA) and protoporphyrin but no nucleus. The reticulocyte count is used to assess the response of the bone marrow to blood loss, hemolysis, and replacement therapy for the treatment of anemia. Healthy marrow produces and releases reticulocytes in response to the need for increased oxygen-carrying capacity.

Vitamin B_{12}. Decreased serum vitamin B_{12} levels are associated with megaloblastic anemias.

White Blood Cells. The three morphologically distinct types of WBCs include granulocytes (neutrophils, basophils, and eosinophils), monocytes, and lymphocytes. The WBC count and differential (the relative percentage and absolute numbers of each type of WBC) are used to diagnose a variety of diseases and monitor the response to drug therapy.

Granulocytes

Eosinophils. Eosinophils are WBCs that contain numerous inflammatory mediators. The number of eosinophils is increased in parasitic infections and allergic reactions. Some neoplastic diseases, skin disorders, and collagen-vascular diseases also may increase the number of circulating eosinophils.

Basophils. Basophils have insignificant phagocytic properties and do not increase in number as a result of infectious processes. Rather, basophils form heparin and have a role similar to that of mast cells in immediate hypersensitivity reactions. The number of basophils may increase in chronic hypersensitivity states, systemic mast cell disease, and myeloproliferative diseases.

Neutrophils. Polymorphonuclear cells are mature WBCs. Their precursors, in order of increasing maturity, are myeloblasts, promyelocytes, myelocytes, metamyelocytes, and band neutrophils. A shift to the left in the differential white cell count means significant numbers of neutrophil precursors such as bands are present. Neutrophils are phagocytic cells that engulf and destroy bacteria. The number of neutrophils is increased in infections, tissue necrosis, inflammatory diseases, metabolic disorders, and some leukemias. The number of circulating neutrophils is increased by corticosteroids, exercise, and epinephrine, all of which cause the release of neutrophils from peripheral storage sites. The number of neutrophils is decreased in overwhelming infection and in some bacterial, viral, and protozoal infections. Marrow depressants, liver disease, and some collagen-vascular diseases are associated with decreased numbers of neutrophils.

Lymphocytes. Lymphocytes are WBCs formed in lymphoid tissue throughout the body. Lymphocytes provide humoral, cell-mediated, and cytotoxic immune responses and interact with antigens in the body. T lymphocytes, which are derived from the thymus, provide cell-mediated immunity; B lymphocytes, which are derived from the bone marrow, provide humoral immunity and produce antibodies. Null lymphocytes have neither T cell nor B cell characteristics. The lymphocyte count is increased in viral disease, bacterial diseases such as whooping cough, metabolic conditions, and chronic inflammatory conditions. The lymphocyte count is decreased in immunodeficiency syndromes, severe illnesses, and diseases associated with abnormalities of the lymphatic circulatory system.

The two types of T lymphocytes include the T4 (helper) and T8 (suppressor) lymphocytes. T4 lymphocytes enhance the response of B cells. T4 lymphocytes are profoundly decreased in acquired immunodeficiency syndrome (AIDS). T8 lymphocytes may be increased in hepatitis B, acute mononucleosis, and cytomegaloviral infection. The T4/T8 lymphocyte ratio reverses in diseases associated with altered immunoregulatory function.

Monocytes. Monocytes are the precursors of macrophages. They are in the circulation only briefly before entering body tissues to become macrophages. The monocyte count is increased in some infectious, granulomatous, and collagen-vascular diseases.

Diagnostic Procedure

Bone Marrow Aspiration. Bone marrow is obtained by penetrating the iliac crest or sternum with a large-bore needle and withdrawing a sample of the bone marrow. The sample is smeared and slides are microscopically evaluated for cell-line precursors and iron stores. Bone marrow aspiration is used to diagnose anemias and leukemias.

THE IMMUNOLOGIC SYSTEM ▌

A variety of laboratory tests and procedures are used to evaluate and monitor the immunologic system. The normal immunologic reference values are listed in Table 5-5.

Laboratory Tests

Autoantibodies. Autoantibodies are used in the monitoring and diagnosis of a variety of autoimmune diseases.[21,22]

Antinuclear antibodies. Antinuclear antibodies (ANAs) are frequently associated with systemic lupus erythematosus (SLE), although they may be present in rheumatoid collagen diseases, mixed connective tissue disease, and systemic sclerosis. ANAs are reported as a titer and a pattern of cellular fluorescence. The patterns include the following:

1. *Homogenous*—Diffuse fluorescence throughout the nucleus

| **Table 5-5** | *Adult Immunologic Laboratory Reference Values (Based on Serum Tests)* |

INDEX	CONVENTIONAL UNITS	SYSTÈME INTERNATIONAL D'UNITÉS
Alpha$_1$-antitrypsin	85-213 mg/dl	0.85-2.13 g/L
Alpha-fetoprotein	<10 IU/ml	<7.75 µg/L
Antinuclear antibodies	Negative at 1:8 dilution	
Antinative DNA antibodies	Negative at 1:10 dilution	
Antibodies to Sm	None	
Antibodies to ribonucleoprotein (RNP)	None	
Antibodies to SS-A (Ro)	None	
Antibodies to SS-B (La)	None	
Complement		
C3	83-177 mg/dl	0.83-1.77 g/L
C4	15-45 mg/dl	0.15-0.45 g/L
Total hemolytic (CH$_{50}$)	150-250 U/ml	150-250 U/L
Rheumatoid factor	<30 IU/ml	<30 kIU/L
Uric acid		
Female	2.3-6.6 mg/dl	137-393 µmol/L
Male	3.6-8.5 mg/dl	214-506 µmol/L

From Jordan DC et al: Normal reference laboratory values, *N Engl J Med* 327:718-724, 1992; Sacher RA, McPherson RA: Widmann's clinical interpretation of laboratory tests, ed 10, Philadelphia, 1991, F.A. Davis; Tilkian SM, Conover MB, Tilkian AG: *Clinical implications of laboratory tests*, ed 4, St Louis, 1987, Mosby.

2. *Ring*—Nuclear border fluorescence
3. *Speckled*—Speckled fluorescence throughout the nucleus
4. *Nucleolar*—Fluorescence in the nucleolar area of the nucleus

Anti-DNA antibodies. Anti-DNA antibodies are antibodies against double-stranded DNA (dsDNA) and single-stranded DNA (ssDNA). Anti-dsDNA antibodies are frequently found in patients with SLE.

Extractable nuclear antigens. Antibodies may be present against specific extractable nuclear antigens (ENAs). These antigens include the Smith (Sm), ribonucleoprotein (RNP), SS-A (Ro), SS-B (La), Scl-70, and histone antigens. SLE is associated with high titers of anti-Sm antibodies. Mixed connective tissue disease and SLE are associated with high titers of anti-RNP antibodies. Systemic sclerosis and SLE are associated with high titers of anti-SS-A and anti-SS-B antibodies. Antibodies against histones may be found in patients with drug-induced SLE. Considerable overlap occurs among the diseases associated with these antibodies.

Rheumatoid factor (RF). Antibodies against immunoglobulin G and M may be found in patients with rheumatoid arthritis.

Cold Agglutinins. Cold agglutinins are antibodies that bind to the surface of RBCs.[23] Agglutination occurs when the blood sample is cooled. Cold agglutinins are associated with a variety of infections and inflammatory disorders.

Coombs' Test. The Coombs' test uses an antiserum containing antibodies that act to bridge antibody-coated or complement-coated RBCs. Agglutination occurs when the cells are bridged.

Direct Coombs' test. The direct Coombs' test uses antibodies directed against human proteins (primarily IgG and C_3) to detect whether these proteins are attached to the surface of RBCs. The direct Coombs' test is used to differentiate between immunologic (e.g., autoimmune) and nonimmunologic (e.g., drug-induced) hemolytic anemias.

Indirect Coombs' test. The indirect Coombs' test detects antibodies against human RBCs in the patient's serum. It is used in crossmatching before transfusion.

Complement. The total serum hemolytic complement (CH_{50}) test is used to screen the integrity of the complement system by testing in vitro the reaction of the patient's serum with presensitized sheep erythrocytes. CH_{50} levels decrease with increased autoimmune disease activity.

Complement Components 3 and 4. Components 3 and 4 (C3 and C4) of the complement system are normally found in relatively high quantities in the serum and are used to diagnose and monitor the progress of autoimmune disease activity.[24] The levels of C3 and C4 decrease with increased disease activity.

C-Reactive Protein. C-reactive protein (CRP) is a nonspecific indicator of inflammation. It is acutely elevated in rheumatoid arthritis, acute bacterial infections, and viral hepatitis. It also is sometimes used to differentiate between bacterial and viral meningitis.

Erythrocyte Sedimentation Rate. The ESR is a nonspecific indicator of inflammation. This test measures the rate at which RBCs settle out of mixed venous blood. The rate of settling is influenced by the shape of the RBC and changes on the membrane. It is a nonspecific marker of inflammatory and malignant disease.

Immunoelectrophoresis. Immunoelectrophoresis uses electrophoretic separation and immunodiffusion techniques to separate proteins. It is used to screen for diseases associated with immunoglobulin abnormalities.

Immunoglobulin E. The serum immunoglobulin E (IgE) is elevated in patients with allergic disorders.

Lupus Anticoagulant. The lupus anticoagulant is a circulating immunoglobulin found in patients with autoimmune disease. It prolongs in vitro clotting time by inhibiting phospholipid interactions but is not associated with an increased risk of bleeding in vivo.

Organ-Specific Autoantibodies. Autoantibodies directed against antigens unique to specific organs may be associated with diseases. For example, antibodies may be detected against the thyroid (thyroiditis), RBC membranes (autoimmune hemolytic anemia), platelet membranes (immune thrombocytopenic purpura), glomerular basement membranes (Goodpasture's disease and glomerulonephritis), intrinsic factor (pernicious anemia), and the acetylcholine receptor (myasthenia gravis).

Protein Electrophoresis. Serum protein electrophoresis is used to screen for serum protein abnormalities. The proteins (albumin, α-1 globulin, α-2 globulin, beta globulin, and gamma globulin) are separated by different migration patterns they follow when subjected to an electric field. This test is used in the diagnosis of diseases associated with immunoglobulin abnormalities.

Uric Acid. Uric acid is the end product of purine metabolism. Low serum levels are associated with Wilson's disease and some malabsorption syndromes. High levels are associated with rapid cellular destruction (such as in chemotherapy or malignancies) and disorders of metabolism such as gout.

Veneral Disease Research Laboratory Test. The Venereal Disease Research Laboratory (VDRL) test, used to diagnose syphilis, is sometimes falsely positive in connective tissue disease.

Diagnostic Procedures

Anergy Panel. An anergy panel is used to test the patient's reactivity to a variety of antigens (purified protein derivative antigen, mumps antigen, *Streptococcus* antigen, candidin, *Trichophyton* antigen, histoplasmin). The antigens are injected intradermally and the skin is evaluated for redness and swelling at the injection site. Response to one or more of the antigens indicates a responsive immune system. Response to a specific antigen indicates that the patient has antibodies to a specific antigen.

Scratch or Patch Testing. Scratch testing is used to evaluate patient sensitivity to specific allergens.[25] Each allergen is applied to the skin by scratching the skin. The skin is then evaluated for swelling and redness.

INFECTIOUS DISEASE

A variety of laboratory and diagnostic tests and procedures are used to diagnose infectious disease and monitor the response to drug therapy.

Laboratory Tests

Acid-Fast Stain. The acid-fast stain is used to screen for the presence of *Mycobacterium, Nocardia,* and *Legionella* species in body tissues and fluids. Some oocysts such as *Cryptosporidium* can be detected with the acid-fast stain.

Cerebrospinal Fluid Analysis. The cerebrospinal fluid is analyzed for the presence and quantity of RBCs, WBCs, glucose, and protein. If indicated, stains (Gram's stain, acid-fast stain) and potassium hydroxide and India ink preparations are used to evaluate the fluid. Normally the cerebrospinal fluid is clear, without blood or organisms. The cerebrospinal fluid glucose is normally about two-thirds the serum blood glucose. Viral meningitis is characterized by a negative Gram's stain and normal protein and glucose. Fungal and tuberculous meningitis is characterized by a negative Gram's stain, normal protein, and low glucose. Bacterial meningitis is characterized by cloudy cerebrospinal fluid, increased WBCs, elevated protein, and frequently a positive Gram's stain.

Cold Agglutinins. Cold agglutinins are antibodies that bind to the surface of RBCs and agglutinate when the blood sample is cooled. About 50% of patients with *Mycoplasma pneumoniae* have cold agglutinin titers.

C-Reactive Protein. The CRP is a nonspecific indicator of inflammation. It is acutely elevated in rheumatoid arthritis, acute bacterial infections, and viral hepatitis. It is sometimes used to differentiate between bacterial and viral meningitis.

Culture and Sensitivity Testing. Cultures of body fluids and tissues are obtained to identify the specific infecting organism. The susceptibility to a variety of antibiotics is determined in vitro.

Cytotoxicity Toxin Assays. The presence of some infectious microorganisms is identified by the presence of specific toxins produced by them rather than by identification of the organism itself. For example, *Clostridium difficile* is detected by the presence of a toxin in the stool.

Gram's Stain. The Gram's stain is used to evaluate a body fluid or specimen for the presence of microorganisms. The organisms can then be characterized according to their gram-positive or gram-negative characteristics, type of organism (e.g., cocci, rod), and special characteristics such as chain or cluster formation.

India Ink Preparation. The India ink preparation is used to detect *Cryptococcus neoformans* in a variety of body fluids. The carbons in India ink are unable to penetrate the organism, enabling the microscopic identification of the organism by its lack of staining.

Minimal Bactericidal Concentration. The minimal bactericidal concentration (MBC) is the lowest antibiotic concentration that kills at least 99.9% of the bacteria in the original inoculum. It is used to determine the susceptibility of the organism to a variety of antibiotics.

Minimum Inhibitory Concentration. The minimum inhibitory concentration (MIC) is the lowest antibiotic concentration that completely inhibits the visible growth of a microorganism. It is used to determine the susceptibility of the organism to a variety of antibiotics.

Potassium Hydroxide Preparation. Potassium hydroxide (KOH) 10% to 20% is used to detect fungi in body fluids and skin scrapings.

Rapid Plasma Reagin Test. The rapid plasma reagin (RPR) test is used to screen for syphilis. It tests for antibodies against antigens from damaged host cells.

Serologic Tests. Serologic tests are used to identify an antigen or antibody to help diagnose infectious disease and monitor the immunologic response to the microorganism.[26] Acute-phase titers and convalescent titers are sometimes compared. Example of serologic tests include the antistreptolysin-O (ASO) titer, cold agglutinin titers, cryptococcal titers, and hepatitis viral serology.

Venereal Disease Research Laboratory Test. The Veneral Disease Research Laboratory (VDRL) test is the only test authorized for testing of the cerebrospinal fluid for syphilis. It tests for the presence of antibodies against antigens from damaged host cells. The VDRL test is not as sensitive as the RPR test.

Wet Mounts. Wet mounts of body fluid specimens are examined microscopically for the presence of parasites and fungi.

White Blood Cell Count and Differential. The WBC count is often elevated in patients with bacterial and viral infections. A left shift (increased bands and segmented neutrophils) is indicative of bacterial infections. The lymphocyte count may be elevated in viral infections. The eosinophil count may be elevated in parasitic infections. Elderly patients and those with impaired immune systems or very severe infectious diseases may not be able to mount a white cell response to infection.

NEUROLOGIC SYSTEM

The neurologic system is evaluated by several highly specialized diagnostic tests and procedures.

Diagnostic Procedures

Caloric Testing (Calorics). Caloric testing is performed by irrigating the external auditory canal with ice-cold water. Both eyes deviate toward the side of the cold water stimulus if the brainstem is intact. If the cerebral hemispheres are intact, the eyes then rapidly move away from the side of the cold-water stimulus.

Edrophonium (Tensilon) Test. The edrophonium test is used to diagnosis myasthenia gravis and determine whether the maintenance acetylcholinesterase inhibitor dosage is appropriate. Edrophonium is administered parenterally and the muscle strength of the patient is evaluated subjectively.

Electroencephalography. The electroencephalograph (EEG) records the electrical activity of the brain from electrodes attached to the scalp. It is used to diagnose seizures and assess the response to drug therapy.

Electromyography. Electromyography (EMG) evaluates muscle action potential from needles inserted into the muscle. It is used to diagnose muscle disease and evaluate response to therapy.

Nerve Conduction Studies. The rate of nerve conduction is evaluated by stimulating the nerve and recording the rate of conduction to electrodes placed over the muscle. Nerve conduction studies are used to diagnose nerve injuries and neuromuscular disease.

NUTRITIONAL ASSESSMENT

Numerous parameters in addition to height and weight are used to assess the nutritional status of a patient and monitor the response to supplemental or total nutritional replacement therapy.[27-29] Normal reference values for nutritional assessment are listed in Table 5-6.

Laboratory Tests

Albumin. Serum albumin is used as an indicator of visceral protein reserves and nutritional status. Protein malnutrition is associated with a serum albumin level of less than 3.5 mg/dl if liver function is normal.

Bilirubin. Conjugation of bilirubin requires energy. Therefore starvation may cause mild hyperbilirubinemia.

Calcium. Decreased serum albumin decreases total calcium. However, the serum calcium does not reflect total body stores.

Creatinine. The 24-hour urinary excretion of creatinine is used to estimate muscle catabolism. Although serum creatinine is not a useful indicator of nutritional status, very low serum creatinine levels may reflect poor nutritional status.

Glucose. Blood glucose is monitored during nutritional supplementation or total nutritional replacement therapy to assess overall metabolic balance. It is not a useful indicator of nutritional status.

Immunologic Status. Malnutrition may be associated with altered immunologic status. Lymphocyte production may be diminished, resulting in a decreased total lymphocyte count. Patients may not be able to mount an immunologic response to skin test antigens.

Magnesium. Decreased serum albumin levels decrease total magnesium. However, the serum magnesium does not reflect total body stores.

Partial Thromboplastin Time. Poor nutritional status may be associated with inadequate intake of vitamin K, resulting in a deficiency of vitamin K–dependent clotting factors and prolonged clotting time.

Phosphorus. Phosphorus is a metabolic cofactor and intermediate. Refeeding hypophosphatemia may occur in patients with low levels of phosphorus who receive nutritional supplementation or total nutritional replacement therapy.

Transaminases. Starvation compromises cellular membrane integrity and may be associated with increased transaminases (AST and ALT).

Table 5-6	*Adult Nutritional Laboratory Reference Values*		
INDEX	SOURCE	CONVENTIONAL UNITS	SYSTÈME INTERNATIONAL D'UNITÉS
Alanine aminotransferase (ALT)			
Female	S*	7-30 U/L	0.12-0.50 μkat/L
Male	S	10-55 U/L	0.17-0.91 μkat/L
Aspartate aminotransferase (AST)			
Female	S	9-25 U/L	0.15-0.42 μkat/L
Male	S	10-40 U/L	0.17-0.67 μkat/L
Bilirubin			
Direct	S	Up to 0.4 mg/dl	Up to 7 μmol/L
Total	S	Up to 1 mg/dl	Up to 17 μmol/L
Blood urea nitrogen	S	8-25 mg/dl	2.9-8.9 mmol/L
Calcium	S	8.5-10.5 mg/dl	2.1-2.6 mmol/L
Glucose (fasting)	P†	70-110 mg/dl	3.9-5.6 mmol/L
Hemoglobin			
Female	WB‡	12-16 g/dl	7.4-9.9 mmol/L
Male	WB	13-18 g/dl	8.1-11.2 mmol/L
Iron	S	50-150 μg/dl	9-26.9 μmol/L
Magnesium	S	1.5-2.0 mEq/L	0.8-1.3 mmol/L
Partial thromboplastin time, activated (aPTT)	P	24-37 sec	24-37 sec
Phosphorus, inorganic	S	2.6-4.5 mg/dl	0.84-1.45 mmol/L
Protein			
Albumin	S	3.1-4.3 g/dl	31-43 g/L
Total	S	6-8 g/dl	60-80 g/L
Total	U§	<165 mg/day	<0.165 g/day
Transferrin saturation	S	20%-45%	20%-45%

From Jordan CD et al: Normal reference laboratory values, *N Engl J Med* 327:718-724, 1992; Sacher RA, McPherson RA: *Widmann's clinical interpretation of laboratory tests,* ed 10, Philadelphia, 1991, F.A. Davis; Tilkian SM, Conover MB, Tilkian AG: *Clinical implications of laboratory tests,* ed 4, St Louis, 1987, Mosby.
*S, Serum.
†P, Plasma.
‡WB, Whole blood.
§U, Urine.

Transferrin.   Transferrin is an iron transport protein with a shorter half-life than albumin (1 week versus 3 weeks). Therefore serum transferrin responds more quickly to changes in nutritional status than does albumin and is a useful indicator of nutritional status.

Blood Urea Nitrogen.   Blood urea nitrogen (BUN) is a useful indicator of protein breakdown.

Diagnostic Procedures

Anthropometrics.   Comparative measurements of parts of the body are used to assess nutritional status. Parameters such as skinfold thickness of the upper portion of the nondominant arm, mid-upper arm circumference (MUAC), and arm muscle circumference (AMC) are measured to assess nutritional status. In general, a

20% to 40% decrease compared with normal values is associated with moderate malnutrition. A greater than 40% decrease is associated with severe malnutrition.

THE RENAL SYSTEM

A variety of laboratory tests are used to diagnose the renal system and monitor the response to drug therapy. Normal adult reference values are in Table 5-7.

Laboratory Tests

Arterial Blood Gas. The arterial blood gas assesses the acid-base balance and level of ventilation. It is used to diagnose acid-base disturbances and monitor the response to drug and nondrug interventions.

Arterial pH. The arterial pH is a quantitative measure of the degree of acidity or alkalinity of the arterial blood.

Base excess. The base excess is a quantitative measurement of the combined buffering capacity of all body buffering systems, including the bicarbonate system and hemoglobin.

Bicarbonate. The bicarbonate is a quantitative measure of net bicarbonate production and elimination.

Table 5-7	*Adult Renal Laboratory Reference Values*		
INDEX	**SOURCE**	**CONVENTIONAL UNITS**	**SYSTÈME INTERNATIONAL D'UNITÉS**
Arterial blood gas			
pH	WB*	7.35-7.45 pH units	7.35-7.45 pH units
P_{CO_2}	WB	35-45 mmHg	4.7-6.0 kPa
P_{O_2}	WB	75-100 mmHg	10-13.3 kPa
Bicarbonate	WB	22-26 mEq/L	22-26 mmol/L
Oxygen saturation	WB	96%-100%	0.96-1.00
Base excess	WB	-2 to $+2$	
Calcium	S†	8.5-10.5 mg/dl	2.1-2.6 mmol/L
Carbon dioxide content	S	24-30.9 mEq/L	24-30.9 mmol/L
Chloride	S	100-108 mEq/L	100-108 mmol/L
Magnesium	S	1.5-2.0 mEq/L	0.8-1.0 mmol/L
Phosphorus	S	2.6-4.5 mg/dl	0.85-1.45 mmol/L
Potassium	S	3.5-5.0 mEq/L	3.5-5.0 mmol/L
Sodium	S	135-145 mEq/L	135-145 mmol/L
Specific gravity	U‡	1.001-1.030	
Urine pH	U	4.8-7.8 pH units	

From Jordan CD et al: Normal reference laboratory values, *N Engl J Med* 327:718-724, 1992; Sacher RA, McPherson RA: *Widmann's clinical interpretation of laboratory tests*, ed 10, Philadelphia, 1991, F.A. Davis; Tilkian SM, Conover MB, Tilkian AG: *Clinical implications of laboratory tests*, ed 4, St Louis, 1987, Mosby.
*WB, Whole blood.
†S, Serum.
‡U, Urine.

Carbon dioxide tension. The partial pressure of dissolved carbon dioxide (PCO_2) is a quantitative measure of net carbon dioxide production and elimination.

Oxygen saturation. The oxygen saturation of the blood (SO_2) is a quantitative measurement of the percent of hemoglobin combined with oxygen. It can be measured noninvasively with pulse oximetry.[30]

Oxygen tension. The partial pressure of oxygen dissolved in the blood (PO_2) is a quantitative measure of oxygen concentration.

Creatinine. Creatinine is filtered by glomerular filtration and is therefore a useful indicator of renal function.

Electrolytes. The serum electrolytes include calcium, chloride, magnesium, phosphorus, potassium, and sodium. The serum concentration of these electrolytes is quite variable and does not indicate total body electrolyte stores.

Calcium. Serum calcium is used to assess calcium metabolism and screen for and evaluate the response to therapy in bone tumors, primary and secondary hyperparathyroidism and hypoparathyroidism, renal failure, and acute pancreatitis. Free and protein-bound calcium are present in the serum; however, only protein-bound calcium is measured. Therefore serum calcium results must be interpreted to take into account the serum albumin (0.8 mg/dl should be added to the measured serum calcium for every 1 gm/dl decrease in serum albumin).

Chloride. Chloride is an extracellular electrolyte. Serum chloride is increased in renal tubular acidosis and primary hyperparathyroidism. It is decreased by the administration of drugs such as thiazide and loop diuretics and prednisone.

Magnesium. Magnesium is an intracellular electrolyte. Serum magnesium is used in the assessment of magnesium deficiency and for monitoring of replacement therapy.

Phosphorus. Phosphorus is present in bone (about 85% of the total) and skeletal muscle (about 10% of the total). The serum phosphorus concentration is always in a 1:1 ratio with the serum calcium concentration. Serum phosphorus is used in the diagnosis of hypoparathyroidism and the assessment of bone metabolism.

Potassium. Potassium is an intracellular electrolyte. The serum concentration is sensitive to changes in acid-base status. Serum potassium is increased in acidosis, dehydration, and renal insufficiency and with the administration of some drugs such as spironolactone. It is decreased in overhydration and alkalosis and with the administration of drugs such as steroids, amphotericin, and lithium carbonate.

Sodium. Sodium is an extracellular electrolyte used to assess water and sodium balance. Serum sodium is increased in dehydration. It is decreased in Addison's disease and by diuretic administration, dilution in ascites, congestive heart failure, renal insufficiency, and excessive water intake.

Gram's Stain and Culture. Normal urine contains no bacteria or yeasts. Bacteria is present in urinary tract infections and pyelonephritis. The Gram's stain and culture are used to identify the etiology of the infection and monitor the response to drug therapy. Yeasts are found in the immunocompromised host and sometimes are associated with broad-spectrum antibiotic therapy.

Osmolality. The urine and serum osmolalities are measured and compared to assess the ability of the kidneys to concentrate the urine. The normal urine-to-serum osmolality ratio is 1:3. Ratios less than 1:1 indicate distal tubular disease. Ratios greater than 1:1 indicate glomerular disease.

Blood Urea Nitrogen. Blood urea nitrogen (BUN), the end product of protein metabolism, is excreted by glomerular filtration. Although it is used as an indicator of renal function, it is less reliable than the serum creatinine because some of the urea diffuses back into the renal tubular cells after filtration. In addition, liver function and protein intake influence the production of BUN.

Urinary Sodium. The urinary sodium is used to differentiate between renal failure from prerenal etiologies (such as dehydration) and from parenchymal renal insufficiency. In renal disease the kidney is unable to conserve sodium, resulting in elevated urine sodium levels. Urinary sodium also is used to diagnose the syndrome of inappropriate antidiuretic hormone secretion (SIADH); in SIADH the serum sodium is low but the urine sodium is elevated.

Urine Toxicology. Urinalysis is used to detect the presence of drugs in patients with suspected drug overdoses, patients experiencing altered mental status, and patients in drug-rehabilitation programs.

Urinalysis. Urinalysis also is used to screen for renal and nonrenal disease and monitor the response to drug and nondrug therapy.[31,32] The urinalysis consists of macroscopic assessment, chemical screening by dipstick, and microscopic assessment of the urine sediment. Quantitative analyses are performed when indicated.

Dipstick screening. Multiple-reagent strips are used to determine the urinary pH and specific gravity and screen for the presence of bilirubin, blood, glucose, ketones, leukocyte esterase, nitrites, pH, protein, and urobilinogen.

Bilirubin. Bilirubin is not normally present in the urine. It is excreted in the urine in the presence of severe liver disease or obstructive biliary disease. The urine appears dark yellow to brown if bilirubin is present.

Blood. Blood is not normally present in the urine. The urine may be visibly bloody or blood may be found on microscopic or dipstick exam. A variety of renal and nonrenal diseases, including urinary tract infections, renal stones, sickle cell disease, glomerulonephritis, and malignant hypertension, are associated with blood in the urine.

Glucose. Glucose is not normally present in the urine. Urine glucose may be present in diabetes mellitus.

Ketones. Ketones are not normally present in the urine. Urinary ketones may be present before serum ketones are detectable in diabetic ketoacidosis and may be found in patients who are dieting or are malnourished.

Leukocyte esterase. Leukocyte esterase is not normally present in the urine. This enzyme is present in WBCs and may be found in the urine during urinary tract and vaginal infections.

Nitrites. Nitrites are not normally present in the urine. *Escherichia coli* converts dietary nitrates to nitrites. Urinary nitrites are associated with *E. coli* urinary tract infections but may only be found if the urine is retained in the bladder for at least 4 hours.

pH. The urinary pH reflects the overall acid-base balance of the body and the kidneys' ability to handle acids and bases. The formation of kidney stones is pH dependent. An alkaline pH (pH greater than 7.0) is commonly associated with the presence of urea-splitting organisms such as *Proteus mirabilis*.

Protein. Protein may be normally present in the urine (as much as 0.5 g/day). Urinary protein is increased in a variety of renal diseases.

Specific gravity. The specific gravity reflects the ability of the kidneys to concentrate urine and the overall state of hydration. The greater the concentration of the urine, the higher the specific gravity.

Urobilinogen. Urobilinogen is not normally present in the urine. It may be excreted in the urine in the presence of severe liver disease or obstructive biliary disease.

Macroscopic assessment

Color. Freshly voided urine is normally pale yellow. Normal urine may range in color from nearly colorless if very dilute to orange if very concentrated.

Turbidity. Freshly voided urine is normally clear. The urine is turbid if bacteria, WBCs, RBCs, yeast, or crystals are present.

Microscopic assessment. The microscopic evaluation assesses the urinary sediment obtained by centrifugation for a variety of casts, cells, and crystals.

Casts. Urinary casts, sometimes known as the *poor man's renal biopsy,* are objects formed and molded within renal tubules. They are cylindrical and composed mostly of protein and cells. They may be convoluted (spiral) if formed in distal convoluted tubules, broad if formed in dilated collecting ducts, and narrow if formed in narrow lumens.

BILE CASTS. Bile casts are acellular casts that contain bile. They are associated with liver disease.

GRANULAR CASTS. Granular casts are acellular casts that have a granular appearance. They are associated with renal and viral disease and exercise.

HEMOGLOBIN CASTS. Hemoglobin casts are acellular casts that contain hemoglobin. They are associated with hemolytic anemias.

HYALINE CASTS. Hyaline casts are acellular casts that consist of a protein matrix. An occasional hyaline cast may normally be present; however, the number of hyaline casts increases with renal disease.

MIXED CELLULAR CASTS. Mixed cellular casts may contain RBCs, WBCs, and renal tubular epithelial cells. These casts are associated with mixed tubular and interstitial renal diseases.

RED BLOOD CELL CASTS. RBC casts are formed if the glomerular basement membrane is damaged. They may be found in acute and focal glomerulonephritis, lupus nephritis, and trauma.

RENAL TUBULAR EPITHELIAL CELL CASTS. Renal tubular epithelial cell casts are found in diseases such as hepatitis and cytomegaloviral infection that are associated with destruction of the tubular epithelium.

WAXY CASTS. Waxy casts are acellular casts that are formed by the breakdown of cellular casts. They are associated with chronic renal disease.

WHITE BLOOD CELL CASTS. WBC casts are associated with interstitial renal inflammation and are found in pyelonephritis.

Cells

RED BLOOD CELLS. Normally, as many as two RBCs per high power field may be present in the urine. The number of RBCs in the urine increases with urinary tract infections, stones, tumors, and strenuous exercise.

RENAL TUBULAR EPITHELIAL CELLS. Renal tubular epithelial cells, shed from the renal tubules, are normally present in the urine.

SQUAMOUS EPITHELIAL CELLS. Squamous epithelial cells are normally present in the urine. They are shed from the urethra and vagina.

WHITE BLOOD CELLS. Normally, as many as five neutrophils per high power field may be found in the urine. The number of WBCs in the urine increases with renal and urinary tract disease and strenuous exercise.

Crystals. Crystals are found in acidic and alkalotic urine. All crystals of pathologic importance are found in acidic urine. Amorphous phosphate crystals and triple phosphate crystals are normal crystals found in alkaline urine. Amorphous urate crystals, calcium oxalate, and uric acid crystals are normal crystals found in acidic urine. A variety of pathologic crystals may be found in alkaline urine.

BILIRUBIN CRYSTALS. Bilirubin crystals are reddish-brown needles, plates, and cubes associated with jaundice and bilirubinemia.

CHOLESTEROL CRYSTALS. Cholesterol crystals are flat plates with notched corners that are associated with the nephrotic syndromes.

CYSTEINE CRYSTALS. Cysteine crystals are hexagonal plates that are associated with congenital cystinuria.

LEUCINE CRYSTALS. Leucine crystals are round, oily-appearing crystals that are associated with severe hepatic disease.

TYROSINE CRYSTALS. Tyrosine crystals are fine needles grouped in sheaves that are associated with severe hepatic disease.

Diagnostic Procedures

Intravenous Pyelogram. The intravenous pyelogram (IVP) is a test used to visualize the entire urinary tract.[33] It uses a parenteral contrast medium that is cleared by glomerular filtration. IVP is used to detect ureteral obstruction, masses, tumors, and cysts.

Retrograde Pyelography. Retrograde pyelography is used to visualize the urine-collecting systems independent of renal function. Contrast media are instilled through a catheter placed in the bladder.

THE RESPIRATORY SYSTEM ▮

A variety of laboratory tests and diagnostic procedures are used to diagnose respiratory diseases and monitor the response to drug therapy.

Laboratory Tests

Arterial Blood Gas. The arterial blood gas is used to assess the acid-base balance and level of ventilation, diagnose acid-base disturbances, and monitor the response to drug and nondrug interventions. Refer to pp. 116-117 for a discussion of the components of the arterial blood gas.

Sputum Analysis. Sputum analysis is used to screen for disease and monitor the response to drug and nondrug therapy. It consists of macroscopic and microscopic assessments.

Macroscopic assessment

Color. The mucus is normally mucoid and clear. Purulent sputum contains pus and is associated with bacterial infection. Uniformly rusty-appearing purulent sputum is indicative of pneumococcal pneumonia. Bright red streaks in viscid sputum are indicative of *Klebsiella* pneumonia. Greenish-black sputum is indicative of gram-negative bacilli infection.

Odor. Normal sputum is odorless. Foul-smelling sputums are indicative of bacterial infections.

Viscosity. Normal sputum is thin and watery. Very thick, sticky, tenacious sputum is found in asthmatic patients.

Volume. Very little sputum is produced normally. The volume of sputum is increased in a variety of diseases, including bronchitis, pneumonia, and tuberculosis.

Microscopic assessment

Charcot-Leyden crystals. Charcot-Leyden crystals are masses of eosinophils.

Curschmann's spirals. Curschmann's spirals are casts of small bronchi and are found in diseases associated with bronchial obstruction such as asthma.

Eosinophils. Eosinophils are present in asthma and other hypersensitivity reactions.

Neutrophils. Neutrophils are found in bacterial and fungal pneumonia and chronic bronchitis.

Diagnostic Procedures

Bronchoscopy. Bronchoscopy is used to visualize the tracheobronchial tree. A flexible bronchoscope is introduced into the tracheobronchial tree through the nose, mouth, or endotracheal or tracheotomy tube. Samples of fluid and tissue may be obtained for Gram's stain, culture, and cytology.[34]

Chest Radiography. Chest x-ray films are commonly taken to aid in the diagnosis of pulmonary and cardiac disease and assess the response to drug and nondrug interventions.[35]

Pulmonary Function Testing. Pulmonary function testing is used to diagnose pulmonary disease, monitor progression of disease, predict response to bronchodilators, and monitor response to drug and nondrug therapy. Pulmonary function testing is performed using a spirometer or body plethysmography. A spirometer detects and records changes in lung volume and flow. Body plethysmography detects changes in intrathoracic pressure and volume. Normal values vary with age, gender, height, and weight. In general, decreases of 20% or more from predicted values are considered significant.

Carbon monoxide diffusing capacity. The carbon monoxide diffusing capacity (DLCO) test is a noninvasive test of lung function. It is an index of the surface area available for gas exchange and is decreased in emphysema, alveolar inflammation, and fibrosis.

Forced expiratory volume in 1 second. The forced expiratory volume in 1 second (FEV_1) is the volume in L of air exhaled during forced exhalation after maximal inspiration. Normally at least 80% of the forced vital capacity is exhaled in the first second. The FEV_1 is used with the forced vital capacity in differentiating between obstructive and restrictive lung disease. An FEV_1 of less than 1 L is indicative of significant lung disease.

Forced vital capacity. The forced vital capacity (FVC) is the amount of air in L that can be blown out of the lungs during forced exhalation after maximal inspiration. It is used with the FEV_1 in differentiating between obstructive and restrictive lung disease. The FEV_1/FVC ratio is decreased in obstructive lung disease and normal in restrictive lung disease.

Peak expiratory flow rate. The peak expiratory flow rate (PEFR) measures the forced expiratory flow in L per minute. It is used to monitor the progression and response to therapy of patients with bronchospastic diseases such as asthma. Patients monitor the PEFR at home with small, hand-held peak flow meters. PEFR variability of greater than 30% is indicative of moderate to severe persistent asthma.

Residual volume. The residual volume (RV) is the volume of air remaining in the lungs after forced expiration. It is measured using body plethysmography. RVs are increased in diseases characterized by small airway obstruction.

Tidal volume. The tidal volume (TV) is the volume of air inspired or expired with normal breathing.

Pulse Oximetry. Pulse oximetry is a noninvasive, transcutaneous technique for the assessment of oxygen saturation.

Quantitative Pilocarpine Iontophoresis (Sweat Test). The concentration of sodium in sweat is measured after stimulation of the sweat glands with topical pilocarpine; low-voltage current is applied to aid in the absorption of the pilocarpine. The sweat test is used in the diagnosis of cystic fibrosis.

Ventilation-Perfusion Scanning (V/Q Scanning). Ventilation-perfusion scanning is used to compare ventilation and perfusion. Images of the airways taken after the inhalation of radiolabeled tracers are compared with images of the pulmonary vasculature taken after the injection of contrast agents. Normally, ventilated and perfused areas match. This test is commonly used to identify pulmonary emboli.

SEROUS BODY FLUIDS |

A variety of laboratory and diagnostic tests are used to evaluate serous body fluids. Pleural, pericardial, peritoneal, and synovial body fluids are commonly examined to determine the etiology (infectious, malignant, or inflammatory) of disease and response to drug and nondrug treatment. Exudates occur as a result of direct membrane and capillary damage; transudates occur when fluid leaks from blood vessels.

Laboratory and Diagnostic Tests

Serous fluids are analyzed for gross appearance, specific gravity, cell counts and differential cell counts, protein, LDH, and cytology. Immunologic assays and cultures may be performed if indicated. Exudates typically have a cloudy appearance and greater specific gravity, protein, LDH, and cell counts than do transudates. The fluid/serum protein and fluid/serum LDH ratios are greater in exudates than they are in transudates.

In addition to the above tests, synovial fluid is often evaluated for the presence of crystals.[36] Crystals are characterized by shape, birefringence in polarized light, and location (intracellular or extracellular). Two types of crystals may be found in synovial fluid.

Monosodium Urate Crystals. Monosodium urate crystals are needle shaped, have negative birefringence, and are found intracellularly and extracellularly. They are associated with gout.

Calcium Pyrophosphate Crystals. Calcium pyrophosphate crystals may be rod shaped, needle shaped, or rhombic. They have positive birefringence and are found intracellularly and extracellularly. They are associated with pseudogout.

| SELF-ASSESSMENT QUESTIONS |

1 Which one of the following is a noninvasive test or procedure?
   a. Venipuncture
   b. Angiography
   c. Paracentesis
   d. Ultrasonography
   e. Radionuclide studies

2 Which one of the following procedures uses external magnetic fields to produce finely detailed images?
   a. CT
   b. MRI

    c. PET

    d. SPECT

    e. Doppler echography

3 A patient is found to have an elevated CK-MB, an elevated LDH_1, and a "flipped" LDH ratio. These results are consistent with a diagnosis of which of the following?

    a. Myocardial infarction

    b. Pneumonia

    c. Renal failure

    d. Cerebrovascular accident

    e. Liver failure

4 Radionuclide angiocardiography is also known as which of the following?

    a. Electrocardiography

    b. Lymphoscintigraphy

    c. Multiple gated acquisition scanning

    d. Echocardiography

    e. Electrophysiology

5 Metyrapone does which of the following?

    a. Stimulates cortisol synthesis

    b. Inhibits production of antidiuretic hormone

    c. Inhibits production of VMA

    d. Increases urine aldosterone

    e. Inhibits cortisol synthesis

6 Which one of the following tests is used to assess hepatic synthetic function?

    a. Lactic dehydrogenase

    b. Serum albumin

    c. Aspartate aminotransferase

    d. Gamma-glutamyl transpeptidase

    e. Total bilirubin

7 A schistocyte is which of the following?

    a. A red blood cell fragment

    b. A red blood cell with a dark center surrounded by a light ring

    c. A red blood cell shaped like a rod

    d. A red blood cell with evenly distributed spicules

    e. A red blood cell with fragments of nuclear DNA

8 Which one of the following is a laboratory test for fungal skin infections?

    a. Rapid plasma reagin test

    b. Veneral Disease Research Laboratory test

    c. Potassium hydroxide preparation

    d. White blood cell count with differential

    e. Cold agglutinin titer

9 Which one of the following is a quantitative measure of combined body buffering systems?

    a. PCO_2

    b. Serum bicarbonate

    c. Oxygen saturation

d. Base excess

e. Serum creatinine

10 The macroscopic evaluation of sputum includes all of the following EXCEPT:

a. Color

b. Viscosity

c. Volume

d. Odor

e. Gram's stain

REFERENCES

1. Jordan CD et al: Normal reference laboratory values, *N Engl J Med* 327:718-724, 1992.
2. Sacher RA, McPherson RA: *Widmann's clinical interpretation of laboratory tests,* ed 10, Philadelphia, 1991, F.A. Davis.
3. Tilkian SM, Conover MB, Tilkian AG: *Clinical implications of laboratory tests,* ed 4, St Louis, 1987, Mosby.
4. Marshall T, Williams J, Williams KM: Electrophoresis of serum isoenzymes and proteins following acute myocardial infarction, *J Chromatogr* 569:323-345, 1991.
5. Technology Subcommittee of the Working Group on Critical Care: Hemodynamic monitoring: a technology assessment, *Can Med Assoc J* 145:114-121, 1991.
6. Taylor BC, Sheffer DB: Understanding techniques for measuring cardiac output, *Biomed Instrum Technol* 24:188-197, 1990.
7. American College of Cardiology/American Heart Association Task Force on Assessment of Diagnostic & Therapeutic Cardiovascular Procedures: ACC/AHA guidelines for the clinical application of echocardiography, *J Am Coll Clin Cardiol* 16:1505-1528, 1990.
8. Drew BJ: Bedside electrocardiographic monitoring: state of the art for the 1990's, *Heart Lung* 20:610-623, 1991.
9. Goldschlager N, Sox HC, Jr.: The diagnostic and prognostic value of the treadmill exercise test in the evaluation of chest pain, in patients with recent myocardial infarction, and in asymptomatic individuals, *Am Heart J* 116:523-535, 1988.
10. Sue DY, Wasserman K: Impact of integrative cardiopulmonary exercise testing on clinical decision making, *Chest* 99:981-992, 1991.
11. Kramer EL: Lymphoscintigraphy: radiopharmaceutical selection and methods, *Nucl Med Biol* 17:57-63, 1990.
12. Weissleder R, Thrall JH: The lymphatic system: diagnostic imaging studies, *Radiol* 172:315-317, 1989.
13. Gibbons RJ: Rest and exercise radionuclide angiography for diagnosis in chronic ischemic heart disease, *Circulation* 84(suppl 1):I93-I99, 1991.
14. Bayer MF: Effective laboratory evaluation of thyroid status, *Med Clin North Am* 75:1-26, 1991.
15. Donald RA: The assessment of pituitary function, *Clin Biochem* 23:23-30, 1990.
16. Tygstrup N: Assessment of liver function: principles and practice, *J Gastroenterol Hepatol* 5:468-482, 1990.
17. Sallie R, Tredger JM, Williams R: Drugs and the liver. Part 1: Testing liver function, *Biopharm Drug Dispos* 12:251-259, 1991.
18. Maglinte DDT, Torres WE, Laufer I: Oral cholecystography in contemporary gallstone imaging: a review, *Radiol* 178:49-58, 1991.
19. Romano TJ, Dobbins JW: Evaluation of the patient with suspected malabsorption, *Gastroenterol Clin North Am* 18:467-483, 1989.
20. Quigley EMM: Intestinal manometry—technical advances, clinical limitations, *Dig Dis Sci* 37:10-13, 1992.
21. Carsons S: Newer laboratory parameters for the diagnosis of rheumatic disease, *Am J Med* 85(Suppl 4A):34-38, 1988.

22. Mackenzie AH: Differential diagnosis of rheumatoid arthritis, *Am J Med* 85(Suppl 4A):2-11, 1988.
23. Silverman GJ, Chen PP, Carson DA: Cold agglutinins: specificity, idiotypy and structural analysis, *Chem Immunol* 48:109-125, 1990.
24. Atkinson JP: Complement deficiency, *Am J Med* 85(Suppl 6):45-47, 1988.
25. Guerin B, Watson RD: Skin tests, *Clin Rev Allergy* 6:211-227, 1988.
26. Weinstein AJ, Farkas S: Serologic tests in infectious disease, *Med Clin North Am* 62:1099-1117, 1978.
27. Habicht J-P, Pelletier DL: The importance of context in choosing nutritional indicators, *J Nutr* 120:1519-1524, 1990.
28. Sauberlich HE: Implications of nutritional status on human biochemistry, physiology, and health, *Clin Biochem* 17:132-142, 1984.
29. Starker PM: Nutritional assessment of the hospitalized patient, *Adv Nutr Res* 8:109-118, 1990.
30. Clark JS et al: Noninvasive assessment of blood gases, *Am Rev Resp Dis* 145:220-232, 1992.
31. Cushner HM, Copley JB: Review: back to basics: the urinalysis: a selected national survey and review, *Am J Med Sci* 297:193-196, 1989.
32. Haber MH: Quality assurance in urinalysis, *Clin Lab Med* 8:431-447, 1988.
33. Hattery RR et al: Intravenous urographic technique, *Radiol* 167:593-599, 1988.
34. Shure D: Transbronchial biopsy and needle aspiration, *Chest* 95:1130-1138, 1989.
35. Krone KD, Weiner SA: Interpreting chest films, *Hosp Med* 22(10):205-207, 210, 215-218, 220-222, 225-227, 231, 1987.
36. McCarty DJ: Crystal identification in human synovial fluids, *Rheum Dis Clin North Am* 14:253-267, 1988.

CHAPTER 6

The Patient Case Presentation

LEARNING OBJECTIVES

1   List each component of the patient case presentation.
2   State the appropriate sequence for presenting the patient case presentation.
3   Given specific patient information, identify its appropriate location in the patient case presentation.
4   Identify the appropriate sequence for presenting laboratory and diagnostic test results.

PATIENT information, including the history, physical examination, medication history, laboratory reports, and progress reports, is available from a variety of documented and undocumented sources. Efficient organization, summarization, documentation, and presentation of this scattered and sometimes complex patient-specific information are difficult without a universally accepted organizational structure. The structured patient case presentation is the accepted tool for documenting and communicating patient information (Figure 6-1). Health care professionals document and verbally communicate patient information for various members of the health care team using a structured patient case format. For example, primary care providers use the structured patient case format to communicate patient information to consultants.

The structured patient case presentation also is an important teaching tool. In the teaching environment the student or trainee verbally presents the patient case to a preceptor or more experienced clinician. The student or trainee learns to organize and present the patient information, and the preceptor uses the details of the case (as presented) to assess the student's understanding of the case and as a starting point for teaching discussions.

COMPONENTS OF THE PATIENT CASE PRESENTATION |

The patient case presentation consists of a summary of all the information known about the patient. The presentation may be considered an up-to-date "snapshot" that provides a complete picture of the patient at admission or first contact for the current medical problem; it provides a thorough summary of the patient's progress to date (Box 6-1).[1-3] Every detail cannot be presented. The person presenting the patient case is responsible for the identification and selection of pertinent details and salient information. The presentation provides all the information needed to understand the patient case but spares the listener a barrage of duplicate, trivial, and irrelevant information.

By convention, each component of the patient case presentation is known by an abbreviation (Table 6-1). These abbreviations are used not only to document the

General Information and Chief Complaint: CW is a 28-year-old white female who presented to her local medical doctor on 10-21-97 with a chief complaint of "I have a rash."

History of Present Illness: CW complains of an itchy rash that started yesterday. She first noticed the rash on her chest and stomach yesterday morning; the rash spread to her arms and legs last night. She couldn't sleep last night because of the itching. She felt warm but did not take her temperature. She relates that she started taking co-trimoxazole (Bactrim) 2 days ago for a urinary tract infection. She is not taking any other medication and has not used any new soaps, detergents, perfumes, or cosmetics.

Past Medical History: She is status post a fractured left tibia at the age of 7 years and an appendectomy at the age of 12 years.

Family History: Her mother is alive and well at the age of 49 years. Her father is alive and well at the age of 51 years; he was recently diagnosed with hypertension. She has three brothers aged 26, 24, and 17 years; all are alive and well.

Social History: CW has a tobacco smoking history of half a pack per day for the past 14 years (a 7 pack-year history). She drinks three to four beers every weekend and has done so for the past 10 years. She denies the use of recreational drugs.

Medication History: CW has no known drug allergies or adverse drug reactions. She started taking Bactrim DS one tablet twice daily on 10-19-97 for a presumed urinary tract infection. Her first dose was at 10 p.m. on 10-19-97. She took one in the morning and evening on 10-20-97 but did not take this morning's dose. She uses no other medication routinely and cannot remember the last time she took a prescription drug.

Review of Systems: As per the HPI.

Physical Examination: CW is a pleasant, well-developed, well-nourished WF in no obvious distress. Her vital signs include a blood pressure of 128/72 mmHg, a heart rate of 88 beats per minute, and a respiratory rate of 10 breaths per minute. Her oral temperature was 99.2° F. She is 5′4″ tall and weighs 52 kg. She has a diffuse maculopapular rash on her trunk and extremities, including the palms of her hands and the soles of her feet. The lesions are red and flat and range in size from a few mm to several large confluent areas (1.5 by 2 cm) on the abdomen and back. The rest of the examination is within normal limits.

Labs: The serum electrolytes were sodium 140 mEq/L, chloride 108 mEq/L, potassium 4.2 mEq/L, and carbon dioxide content 26 mEq/L. The blood urea nitrogen was 10 mg/dl, and the serum creatinine was 1.1 mg/dl. The hemoglobin was 14 g/dl and the hematocrit was 45%. The white blood cell count was 8500 cells/mm^3 with 53% polys, 5% bands, 27% lymphocytes, and 15% eosinophils. The platelets were adequate. The AST was 34 U/L, the ALT was 29 U/L, the alkaline phosphatase was 45 U/L, the lactic dehydrogenase was 240 U/L, the GGT was 16 U/L, the total bilirubin was 0.8 mg/dl, and the albumin was 5.2 g/dl. Urinalysis from 10-19-97 showed greater than 10^6 organisms per ml; the culture was positive for *E. coli*.

Problem List and Initial Plans

Problem #1—Maculopapular urticarial rash; probably drug related. Discontinue the Bactrim DS and avoid sulfonamide-containing medications. Treat with cool water compresses and lukewarm water baths. Consider an oral antihistamine if the itching persists. Consider a short course of oral corticosteroids if rash does not resolve.

Problem #2—*E. Coli* urinary tract infection. Begin amoxicillin 250 mg every 8 hours for 7 days. Alternatives include amoxicillin-clavulanic acid, cephalosporins, and quinolones. Reculture if still symptomatic.

Problem #3—Tobacco smoker. Counsel regarding consequences of smoking and smoking cessation options.

Problem #4—Status post fractured left tibia. Inactive problem.

Problem #5—Status post appendectomy. Inactive problem.

FIGURE 6-1 *Example of a Patient Case Presentation.* The patient case presentation is a verbal summary of patient information.

| Box 6-1 | *Components of the Patient Case Presentation* |

1. General information at the time of admission or first contact
   a. Name, age, race, gender
   b. Date of admission or first contact
2. Chief complaint
3. History of present illness
4. Past medical history
5. Family history
6. Social history
7. Medication history
8. Review of systems
9. Physical examination
   a. General descriptive statement
   b. Vital signs
      1. Blood pressure
      2. Heart rate
      3. Temperature
      4. Respiratory rate
   c. Pertinent positive and negative findings on physical examination
10. Pertinent positive and negative laboratory and diagnostic test results
    a. Serum electrolytes (sodium, chloride, carbon dioxide content), creatine (Cr), blood urea nitrogen (BUN), blood sugar (BS)
    b. Complete blood count (CBC), including white blood cell (WBC) count, differential, hemoglobin (Hgb), hematocrit (HCT), and platelets (PLTS)
    c. Liver function tests (LFTs)
    d. Urinalysis (UA)
    e. Chest x-ray (CXR) film
    f. Electrocardiogram (ECG)
    g. Other test results
11. Patient problem list and initial plans
12. Patient progress
13. Discharge data (if applicable)
    a. Final diagnosis
    b. Discharge medications
14. Plans for follow-up

patient case information in the medical record but also are sometimes used in the presentation of the patient case. For example, clinicians commonly say "HPI" instead of "history of present illness" and "PMH" instead of "past medical history."

The sequence of presentation is important (Box 6-2). The sequence is designed to provide a logical flow of information, starting with information about the current medical issue and finishing with an update on the patient's progress. Listeners tend to relax and listen to the information being presented if they recognize that the information is presented in a generally accepted format. Details may be overlooked if the listener must piece the patient information together or worry about missing important details of the case.

General Patient Information

The general patient information includes the date and time of admission to the hospital or arrival at the clinic or office and the patient's name, age, race, and gender.

Table 6-1	*Patient Case Abbreviations*		
ABBREVIATION	MEANING	ABBREVIATION	MEANING
CC	Chief complaint	ROS	Review of systems
HPI	History of present illness	MedHx	Medication history
PMH	Past medical history	PE	Physical examination
FH	Family history	Labs	Laboratory and diagnostic test results
SH	Social history		

Chief Complaint

The chief complaint (CC) is the reason or reasons the patient is seeking medical care. It is presented and documented in the patient's own words, which provides a better sense of the patient's experiences and conveys a better understanding of the patient's perception of the urgency and severity of the problem. The patient's words also provide important information regarding level of education and medical sophistication. For example, few patients would present a CC of "myocardial infarction." More likely, they would complain of heavy, squeezing, or crushing chest pain and discomfort. However, patients with chronic disease and repeated contact with the health care system and patients who are health care professionals may use sophisticated medical terminology.

Some patients may not provide a CC. If a patient is comatose or otherwise unable to communicate, no CC is presented during the patient case presentation or documented in the medical record. However, the patient's family or friends may be able to describe the patient's problem; this information is sometimes presented as the CC with a notation of the person supplying the information (e.g., "The patient's wife found him unconscious on the living room floor"). Patients who have been referred for specific tests, procedures, and evaluations may not offer a CC. In this case the CC may be presented as "referred for cardiac catheterization," for example.

History of Present Illness

The history of present illness (HPI) is a narrative that describes the current medical problem. All characteristic details such as specific symptoms, the way the problem began or was first recognized by the patient, duration, test results from previous evaluations, activities and treatments that ease and worsen the problem, and past experiences with the problem are included in the HPI. Pertinent data from previous hospitalizations and interventions such as dates of admission and discharge, results of tests and diagnostic procedures, medications used to treat the problem, and physiologic data such as serum creatinine and arterial blood gases also are included.

The HPI is presented in a logical and temporally appropriate sequence. Enough detail should be presented to describe the problem, but excessive and repetitive detail should be avoided. For example, information presented about pain includes location, time of onset, quality (sharp, dull), severity (mild, moderate, severe), duration (acute, chronic), location of any radiating pain, and interventions that ease and worsen the pain (elevation, warmth, cold, food, water, medications).

Risk factors for diseases and conditions such as myocardial infarction, hypertension, diabetes mellitus, and tuberculosis are included in the HPI if the patient

Box 6-2	*Suggested Sequence for Presentation of Information during the Patient Case Presentation*

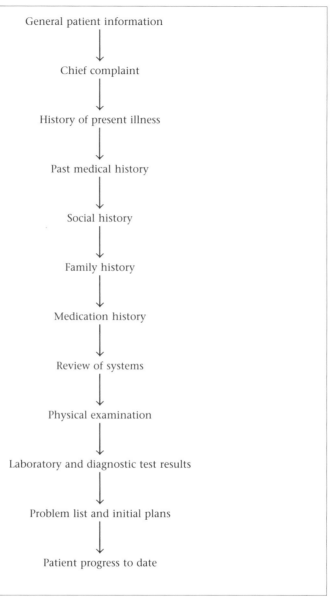

General patient information

↓

Chief complaint

↓

History of present illness

↓

Past medical history

↓

Social history

↓

Family history

↓

Medication history

↓

Review of systems

↓

Physical examination

↓

Laboratory and diagnostic test results

↓

Problem list and initial plans

↓

Patient progress to date

has been diagnosed with one of these diseases or if the CC is suggestive of one. For example, information regarding a family history of cardiac disease and the patient's history of hypertension, smoking, and previous myocardial infarctions is presented if myocardial infarction is suspected.

The HPI also includes pertinent negative patient information—symptoms and complaints the patient might be expected to have given the current complaint but does not. For example, the HPI for a patient complaining of dizziness might include a statement that the patient does not have a history of fever, vomiting, diarrhea, blood in the stool or urine, chest pain, palpitations, or head trauma.

Past Medical History

The past medical history (PMH) includes a brief description of current and previous patient problems unrelated to the present illness. For example, a patient may have hypertension and diabetes but be seeking care for complaints of cough, fever, and chills. The history of hypertension and diabetes is mentioned briefly in the HPI and presented in detail in the PMH.

The PMH includes the approximate dates the problems were first identified and the duration of the problems. It also includes information regarding surgeries and other major medical procedures (e.g., cardiac catheterization, bronchoscopy, skin biopsy). The abbreviation *S/P*, which stands for *status post,* is used to indicate a past event. For example, the PMH may include the following:

> Mild to moderate hypertension for 10 years; insulin-dependent diabetes mellitus for 5 years; glaucoma for 25 years; S/P fractured left tibia in 1979; S/P three vessel CABG [coronary artery bypass graft] in November 1985; S/P T&A [tonsillectomy and adenoidectomy] as a child.

Deciding which information belongs in the HPI and which belongs in the PMH is sometimes difficult. Generally, if details from the patient's PMH directly relate to the current problem, they are included as part of the HPI. For example, if a patient describes a CC of angina, details from the patient's history regarding previous myocardial infarctions and cardiac bypass surgery are included in the HPI.

Social History

The social history (SH) contains information about the patient's use of tobacco, alcohol, and illicit drugs. It also contains information about the patient's occupation, marital status, sexual history, and living conditions.

Tobacco use is quantified in packs per day and pack-years. See page 44 in Chapter 3 for information regarding the way to express a patient's smoking history in pack-years. The interviewer should note whether the patient is currently smoking and the date and reason the patient stopped smoking.

The type, amount, pattern, and duration of alcohol ingestion are described in the SH. For example, alcohol consumption may be described as "a fifth of whiskey daily for the past 15 years" or "a case of beer every weekend for 6 years." The term *social drinking* is sometimes used to describe the drinking habits of patients who do not drink regularly but only if dining out and attending other social occasions. However, because the term is open to wide interpretation, the interviewer should instead quantify the type, amount, pattern, and duration of alcohol ingestion. The date and time of the last drink should be noted for patients who drink regularly.

The use of illicit or so-called recreational or street drugs may be documented in the SH instead of or in place of documenting this information in the medication history. As with the documentation of alcohol use, the amount, pattern, and duration of use of these agents are described in the SH. For example, the interviewer may note that a patient smokes marijuana every weekend and has done so for 8 years or uses crack cocaine daily and has done so for 3 years. As with documentation of the use of alcohol, the date of the last use of these drugs should be noted.

The patient's occupation is documented in the SH. This information is important for both diagnostic reasoning and therapeutic planning. For example, a 40-year history of working in a naval shipyard may be an important piece of information for a patient with pulmonary complaints consistent with mesothelioma. Knowing a patient's work schedule and environment before making decisions regarding the best therapeutic regimen for the patient also may be helpful. For example, the selection of a diuretic as the initial drug treatment for a patient with mild to moderate hypertension may not be the best choice if the patient has a work schedule that precludes frequent rest room breaks. Some jobs such as assembly line factory jobs do not permit much individual privacy; patients with these types of jobs may be reluctant to be seen taking medication. Compliance for these patients may be enhanced by selecting medications with dosing schedules that permit the patient to take the medication in the privacy of the home.

The patient's living conditions are documented in the SH. For example, the interviewer may note that the patient lives at home with a spouse and children or is currently living in a homeless shelter. For patients with physically limiting diseases such as rheumatoid arthritis and emphysema, information regarding the layout of the house is an important part of the SH.

Family History

The family history (FH) consists of a brief summary of the medical histories of the patient's first-degree relatives (parents, siblings, and offspring). Data presented in the FH include information on the status (alive or dead) of the patient's parents, siblings, and children, cause of death and age at death for family members who have died, and current health problems of living family members.

A number of abbreviations and shorthand notations are used for the FH. These abbreviations are not verbally presented but are used to document the FH in the medical record. Common abbreviations include M for mother, F for father, B for brother, and S for sister. An arrow pointing up (↑) indicates the individual is alive; an arrow pointing down (↓) indicates the individual is dead. For example, the notation *M↓ 78(MI)* indicates the patient's mother died at the age of 78 from a myocardial infarction.

The FH may be detailed and well documented for several generations if the patient is suspected of having a genetically linked disease. The patient's family pedigree is documented using a set of universally recognized symbols (Figure 6-2). The age of each relative may be noted near the symbol.

Medication History

Most medication histories obtained and documented by nonpharmacist health care professionals lack the detail of those obtained and documented by pharmacists. Therefore the pharmacist should include the detailed information obtained from the patient medication history interview when making patient case presentations. (See Chapter 3 for information regarding the patient medication history and Box 3-4 on p. 43 for specific data included in the medication history.)

Review of Systems

The review of systems (ROS) summarizes all patient complaints not included in the HPI. It typically follows an organ system approach (e.g., head, heart, lung); pertinent positive findings are presented. For example, a patient may have a CC of cough and fever. When asked about other complaints or problems, a patient may note

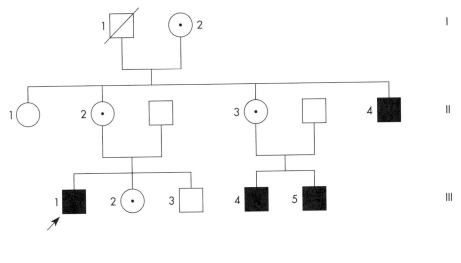

Key

 Unaffected male

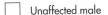

Unaffected female

Affected male

Affected female

Carrier

Deceased

Propositus (the patient that brings the family under study)

FIGURE 6-2 *Family Pedigrees.* Family pedigrees provide information about genetically linked diseases and their transmission across generations. *Roman numerals* indicate generation, and *Arabic numerals* provide patient reference numbers within each generation.

chronic constipation. The HPI describes the CC of cough and fever in detail, but information about the chronic constipation is described in the ROS.

Physical Examination

Presentation of the physical examination (PE) typically begins with a short description of the patient. The patient description helps listeners visualize the patient and begin to anticipate pertinent findings on examination. The listener formulates different impressions and anticipates the presentation of substantially different data from the PE based on the initial patient description. Note the difference in the impressions given by the descriptions of patients A and B:

Patient A is a pleasant, cooperative 48-year-old African-American female in mild respiratory distress.
Patient B is a white female of unknown age who is unconscious and intubated.

The initial description of the patient is followed by a listing of the patient's vital signs, including the blood pressure and heart rate (supine, sitting, or standing as indicated by the patient's initial complaint), respiratory rate, and temperature.

Pertinent positive and negative findings from the PE are presented next (see Chapter 4 for information regarding physical assessment). Pertinent positive findings such as abnormalities found on PE and negative findings such as abnormalities expected to have been found on PE given the patient's complaints or current or potential medical problems that were absent on examination are presented in an organized sequence and format. For example, a logical sequence of presentation of this information is to present the findings from the skin; head, eyes, ears, nose, and throat (HEENT); heart; chest; abdomen; genitalia; and extremities. Findings from the neurologic examination are presented last.

Laboratory and Diagnostic Test Results

Results from laboratory and diagnostic tests and procedures are presented after the findings from the PE (see Chapter 5 for information regarding laboratory and diagnostic tests and procedures). The amount of detail depends on the severity and complexity of the patient's medical problem. In some simple, straightforward patient cases, simply stating that all laboratory findings or all laboratory findings except one specific test such as the chest x-ray film were within normal limits may be sufficient. However, many clinicians find the presentation of all laboratory findings helpful. Students and trainees may be expected to present and comment on every laboratory and diagnostic test and procedure reported for the patient.

No single universally appropriate sequence is available for presenting laboratory and diagnostic test results. However, a common order of sequence is to present the serum electrolytes (sodium, chloride, potassium, carbon dioxide content), glucose, blood urea nitrogen and creatinine first, followed by the complete cell count (white blood cells with differential, hemoglobin, hematocrit, platelets), other electrolytes and serum chemistries, and macroscopic and microscopic urinalysis. Results of additional nonroutine laboratory tests are presented next, followed by a description of electrocardiograms, radiographs, and other diagnostic tests and procedures.

Patient Problem List

The patient problem list and initial diagnostic and therapeutic plans are presented after the presentation of laboratory and diagnostic test results. The patient problem list is a brief listing of the patient's problems, starting with the most acute problem (see Chapter 7 for information regarding problem identification, prioritization, therapeutic planning, and monitoring). Physicians include a list of the differential diagnoses for the problem and an initial plan for treating the problem when presenting the problem list; pharmacists focus on therapeutic planning.

Progress to Date or Hospital Course

All the information presented so far describes the initial presentation of the patient. No additional information is presented if the patient is newly admitted or is being evaluated at an initial clinic visit. However, a great deal more information is available for hospitalized patients and those who have had other clinic or office visits for the same medical problem. This additional information is important for understanding the patient case and should be presented with information about the initial patient presentation in a logical, temporal sequence. For example, presenting every vital sign documented for a patient who has been hospitalized for several days for the management of hypertension is tedious and unnecessary. However, summarizing the blood pressure and heart rate findings in relation to the type of therapy instituted and duration of the specific therapy is appropriate.

Other Information

Additional information beyond that described in this chapter may be presented as part of the patient case presentation if applicable. This information, which may include plans for additional diagnostic procedures and therapeutic interventions, discharge plans, plans for follow-up after discharge from the hospital, and autopsy results, is presented at the end of the patient case presentation.

SELF-ASSESSMENT QUESTIONS

1   A patient had an appendectomy 40 years ago. This information belongs in which section of the patient case?
   a. HPI
   b. PMH
   c. SH
   d. FH
   e. ROS

2   A patient relates smoking four packs of cigarettes a day and doing so for 8 years. This is equivalent to how many pack-years?
   a. 32
   b. 16
   c. 12
   d. 8
   e. 4

3   A patient goes to the local medical doctor with angina. The patient states having several migraine headaches per year. The information about the migraine headaches belongs in which section of the patient case?
   a. HPI
   b. SH
   c. FH
   d. ROS
   e. Laboratory and diagnostic test results

4   Vital signs include all of the following EXCEPT:
   a. Blood pressure
   b. Cardiac output
   c. Temperature
   d. Respiratory rate
   e. Heart rate

5   A patient's 96-year-old mother is alive and well. This information belongs in which section of the patient case?
   a. HPI
   b. PMH
   c. SH

d. FH

e. ROS

6   Which of the following laboratory test results should be presented first?

a. Chest x-ray film

b. Urinalysis

c. Serum electrolytes

d. Electrocardiogram

e. Hemoglobin

7   Which of the following is presented first in the patient case presentation?

a. Patient progress

b. CC

c. PE

d. HPI

e. Medication history

8   Which of the following is presented last in the patient case presentation?

a. Patient progress

b. CC

c. PE

d. HPI

e. Medication history

9   In a family pedigree, what does a closed box with a slash indicate?

a. Unaffected living male

b. Affected living male

c. Unaffected deceased male

d. Affected deceased male

e. Propositus

10   A 42-year-old man is admitted with a suspected myocardial infarction. His risk factors for myocardial infarction (smoking, hypertension, positive family history, hypercholesterolemia, and obesity) are listed in which section of the patient case?

a. HPI

b. PMH

c. SH

d. FH

e. ROS

REFERENCES

1.   Kassirer JP, Kopelman RI: The case presentation: 1. Principles, *Hosp Pract* 23:21, 25-26, 29, 1988.

2.   Kihm JT et al: Quantitative analysis of the outpatient oral case presentation, *J Gen Intern Med* 6:233-236, 1991.

3.   Yurchak PM: A guide to medical case presentations, *Res Staff Phys* 27:109-111, 114-115, 1981.

C H A P T E R 7

Therapeutics Planning

LEARNING OBJECTIVES

1 List the components of the planning process.
2 List the steps involved in the identification of patient problems.
3 Identify subjective and objective patient parameters.
4 List the steps involved in prioritization of patient problems.
5 Prioritize patient problems.
6 List the steps involved in the selection of specific therapeutic regimens.
7 Describe the subjective objective assessment plan (SOAP) format.

PLANNING is the heart of the decision-making process. Effective planning facilitates the selection of appropriate medication regimens for specific patient problems and provides a framework for monitoring patient response to therapy. Planning also incorporates well-thought-out alternative treatment regimens.

The planning process consists of problem identification and prioritization, selection of treatment regimens for each patient problem, and development of an integrated monitoring plan (Box 7-1). Successful planning requires expert knowledge of pharmacotherapeutics, human diseases, physical assessment, and laboratory and diagnostic tests (Figure 7-1). In addition, the pharmacist must be able to determine the way patient factors influence medications and medications influence patient factors. This chapter describes problem identification and prioritization and selection of specific medication regimens; monitoring is discussed in Chapter 8.

PROBLEM IDENTIFICATION

Specific patient problems are identified through evaluation of data obtained from the patient's history, physical examination, laboratory and diagnostic tests, and the medication history acquired by the pharmacist. Subjective and objective findings are identified and evaluated to determine factors that when grouped together are consistent with specific patient problems.

Step 1—Identification of Patient Parameters from the Medical History, Physical Examination, Laboratory and Diagnostic Tests, and the Medication History Acquired by the Pharmacist

The pharmacist should create a working list that includes all subjective and objective parameters. The identification of relevant subjective and objective parameters from the medication history, history of present illness, past medical history, social history, review of systems, physical examination, and laboratory and diagnostic tests requires patience and methodical scrutiny. Subjective parameters include

Box 7-1   *The Planning Process*

1. Problem identification
   Step 1—Identification of subjective and objective patient parameters
   Step 2—Grouping of related parameters
   Step 3—Assessment of the parameters and determination of specific patient problems
2. Problem prioritization
   Step 1—Identification of active problems
   Step 2—Identification of inactive problems
   Step 3—Ranking of the problems
3. Selection of specific therapeutic regimens
   Step 1—Creation of a list of therapeutic options
   Step 2—Elimination of drugs from the list based on patient-specific and external factors
   Step 3—Selection of dosage, route, and duration of therapy
   Step 4—Identification of alternative therapeutic regimens
   Step 5—Creation of a monitoring plan
   Step 6—Monitoring and modification of the regimens as necessary

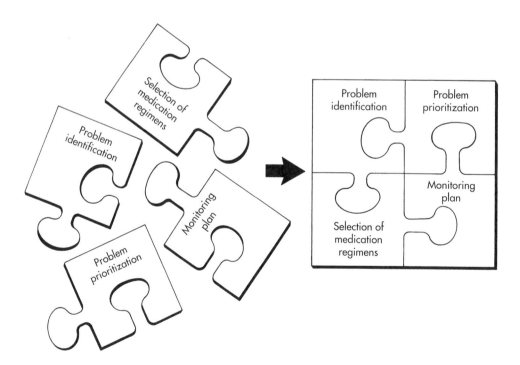

FIGURE 7-1 *Components of Therapeutics Planning.* Therapeutics planning consists of problem identification and prioritization, selection of specific initial and alternative medication regimens for patient problems, and development of a monitoring plan.

Box 7-2 *Common Subjective Parameters*

Anxiety	Headache	Palpitations
Bloating	Heartburn	Pounding pulse
Blood-tinged sputum	Heat intolerance	Rash
Blurred vision	Impotence	Seizures
Breast tenderness	Indigestion	Shortness of breath
Chills	Insomnia	Slurred speech
Cold intolerance	Itching	Sneezing
Confusion	Joint pain	Sore throat
Constipation	Loss of appetite	Syncope
Cramps	Loss of libido	Thirst
Decreased appetite	Muscle aches	Tingling
Depression	Muscle weakness	Tinnitus
Diarrhea	Nasal congestion	Tremor
Difficulty concentrating	Nasal itching	Vertigo
Dry skin	Nausea	Weakness
Dysuria	Nervousness	Wheezing
Fatigue	Numbness	
Flatulence	Pain	

Box 7-3 *Common Objective Parameters*

Height and weight
Vital signs—Temperature, blood pressure, heart rate, respiratory rate
Blood chemistries—Sodium, potassium, chloride, carbon dioxide content, glucose, creatinine, aspartate aminotransferase, alanine aminotransferase, bilirubin, calcium, magnesium, cholesterol, triglycerides, alkaline phosphatase, lactic dehydrogenase, uric acid, urea nitrogen
Blood gases—pH, P_{CO_2}, P_{O_2}, bicarbonate
Blood proteins—Total protein, albumin, complements, immunoglobulins
Hematology—Hemoglobin, hematocrit, mean corpuscular volume, mean corpuscular hemoglobin concentration, red blood cell count, white blood cell count and differential
Urinalysis—Specific gravity, cellular content, protein
Cultures and sensitivities—Blood, urine, sputum, tissue
Serum blood concentrations
Specific organ system tests—Peak expiratory flow rate, forced expiratory volume in 1 second and forced vital capacity (and the ratio of the two), ejection fraction, triiodothyronine, thyroxine, thyroid-stimulating hormone, creatinine clearance
Miscellaneous—Urine output, abdominal girth, number of loose stools per day, input and output

---

coughing, pain, and itching; they can be described but not precisely quantified or measured (Box 7-2). Objective parameters include blood pressure and temperature; they can be precisely quantified or measured (Box 7-3). Physical examination and laboratory and diagnostic parameters are relatively easy to recognize. They are abnormal physical assessment findings and laboratory and diagnostic test results that fall outside the reference range. Subjective parameters may be less obvious and more difficult to identify. Conventionally, parameters such as crackles, edema, and muscle atrophy that are observed by the health care professional during the physical examination but cannot be precisely quantified are considered objective parameters.

Step 2—Creation of Sets of Related Parameters

The pharmacist should evaluate the list of objective and subjective parameters for possible relationships among the parameters and try to determine abnormalities that may be related to one another and may combine to indicate specific patient problems. For example, patient data that include subjective complaints of fever, chills, and productive cough and objective data of leukocytosis with an increased percentage of bands, a chest x-ray film showing right middle lobe consolidation, and sputum positive for gram-positive encapsulated cocci in pairs indicate pneumonia.

Step 3—Creation of a Patient Problem List

The clinical pharmacist should evaluate each group of subjective and objective parameters and determine the specific patient problem or issue. Patient problems include current medical problems such as hypertension, pneumonia, asthma, diabetes, and gastrointestinal bleeding; past medical problems such as a history of migraine headache, hip fracture, deep vein thrombosis, and myocardial infarction; past surgeries such as appendectomy, tonsillectomy, coronary artery bypass grafts, and transurethral resection of the prostate; and issues such as noncompliance, obesity, drug abuse, and allergies. Some pharmacists consider corticosteroid dependency and chronic anticoagulation therapy identifiable problems and separate them from the medical problems that prompted the drug therapy such as steroid-dependent asthma and recurrent thrombophlebitis.

PROBLEM PRIORITIZATION

The second step in the planning process is the prioritization of the patient problem list. Prioritization means ranking patient problems with the most urgent problems on the top of the list and the least urgent problems on the bottom. Prioritization is a way of ordering the relative acuteness of the problems and is not meant to imply a rank ordering of importance or significance to the patient's overall health care needs.

Step 1—Identification of the Patient's Active Problems

Active problems require drug or nondrug intervention. Pneumonia, asthma, congestive heart failure, trauma, cerebrovascular accident, myocardial infarction, and anxiety are active problems.

Step 2—Identification of the Patient's Inactive Problems

Inactive problems are of historical interest only and do not require drug or nondrug intervention. For example, a history of appendectomy, pneumonia 2 years ago, smoking two packs of cigarettes per day until quitting 10 years ago, and sulfa-associated rash are inactive problems.

Step 3—Ranking of the Problems

One approach to problem prioritization is to look at the problem list and determine the problem that if left untreated may result in the most harm to the patient in the shortest amount of time. This problem is ranked as the number one problem. The pharmacist repeats the ranking process with the remaining problems until all are ranked. For example, if the list includes bacterial meningitis, obesity, and a history of a broken leg as a child, the bacterial meningitis is clearly the most life-threatening problem, the history of a broken leg as a child is the least life-threatening problem, and the obesity is active but not immediately life threatening. Another approach is to work from the bottom of the list, determining the problem requiring the least attention. This problem is ranked as the least important problem. The pharmacist repeats the ranking process with the remaining problems until all are ranked. Regardless of the approach used, the active problems are at the top of the list, inactive problems are at the bottom, and active but less acute problems are in the middle. The rank ordering is a rather arbitrary process if the problems all have relatively equal acuity.

Different clinical pharmacists given the same list of patient parameters develop different problem lists. This is not unexpected; no one list is correct. Lists are developed based on the clinical judgment and experience of the practitioner. In addition, because the focus of the pharmacist is on therapeutic issues rather than on differential diagnosis, the pharmacist-generated patient problem list may be similar although not necessarily identical to the problem list generated by other health care professionals.

SELECTION OF SPECIFIC THERAPEUTIC REGIMENS

Selection of specific therapeutic regimens for each patient problem, including initial and alternative medication regimens, takes place after patient problems have been identified and prioritized. Decisions have to be made regarding the most appropriate medication or combination of medications for the management of each problem. The recommendation includes the specific medication, dosage, route of administration, dosage formulation, duration of therapy, and rationale. The general approach is to develop the therapeutic plan for each problem and then integrate the individual plans, making sure that each component of the integrated plan is achievable for the specific patient.

Selection of a specific regimen requires assessment of each patient problem in the context of information known about the patient and external factors. The pharmacist must consider interventions that have and have not worked for the patient in the past, the influence of other patient problems on the proposed medication regimen, and the influence of the proposed regimen on all other patient problems (Box 7-4). For example, a patient who has responded well to a specific decongestant in the past will most likely respond well to the same decongestant in the future. A patient with renal insufficiency is at risk of developing seizures from the accumulation of normeperidine, a renally eliminated metabolite of meperidine. A drug with negative inotropic effects may worsen a patient's congestive heart failure.

External factors to be considered when selecting an optimal therapeutic regi-

Box 7-4	*Factors to Consider when Selecting a Specific Therapeutic Regimen*

Patient-specific factors
    What regimens have effectively managed the problem in the past?
    What regimens have not effectively managed the problem in the past?
    How might other patient problems influence the proposed regimen?
    How might the proposed regimen influence other patient problems?
External factors
    Current "state of the art" therapeutics
    Cost of the proposed therapy
    Formulary limitations

men include the current state-of-the-art therapeutics for managing the specific problem, cost considerations, and limitations imposed by institutional and state formularies. Rarely is any single therapeutic regimen the only possible appropriate regimen; many different regimens may be equally effective for the patient. The decision between equally effective regimens is based on experience and personal preference.

Step 1—Creation of a List of Therapeutic Options for Each Problem

The clinical pharmacist must identify all classes of drugs and possible therapeutic approaches for each problem. At this point, no option should be eliminated for any reason. This step may require review of current pharmacotherapeutics and human disease textbooks or literature searches of the current pharmacy and medical literature. This step becomes easier and more time efficient with practice and experience.

Step 2—Elimination of Therapeutic Options from the List Created in Step 1

The elimination of therapeutic options is based on the comparative effectiveness of the drug; suitability of the drug for the patient given the other patient problems; ability of the patient to comply with the proposed regimen; and other factors such as the effectiveness of previous treatment regimens, cost, and formulary restrictions. The pharmacist must consider the impact of the therapeutic option on other patient problems and the influence of other patient problems on the therapeutic option.

Step 3—Selection of an Appropriate Therapeutic Regimen for Each Problem

Decisions about the most appropriate medication regimen are based on past patient experiences, assessment of the severity of the problem, drug-specific factors such as the therapeutic index of the drug, and specific patient factors such as chronic renal or hepatic disease that may influence the elimination or metabolism of the drug. The recommendation of a regimen includes the specific drug, dosage, route, duration of therapy, and reason the drug was selected.

Step 4—Identification of Alternative Regimens

An important part of the planning process includes anticipation of potential patient problems. A well-constructed plan includes alternative medication regimens

| Box 7-5 | *Guidelines for Altering Initial Drug Therapy* |

If the regimen is ineffective, change the drug if the following are true:
1. The patient received an adequate trial of the drug.
2. The patient received an adequate dosage of the drug.
3. The patient is compliant.

If the regimen is associated with life-threatening side effects, discontinue the drug.

If the patient is not complying with the regimen because of unacceptable side effects, discontinue the drug.

If the patient has non–life-threatening side effects and is willing to continue the drug, minimize the side effects by doing the following:
1. Adjust the dosage of the drug.
2. Change the timing of the doses.

for common potential problems such as the development of an allergy or adverse reaction to the initial therapeutic regimen, lack of desired therapeutic response to the initial therapeutic regimen, and additional patient problems influencing the effectiveness or metabolism of the initial therapeutic regimen. Anticipation of these potential problems allows for the creation of well-thought-out alternative therapeutic plans instead of therapeutic plans hastily chosen after an unanticipated patient problem. For example, therapeutic planning for a patient with newly diagnosed hypertension must include plans for alternative therapeutic regimens if the initial treatment fails to lower the blood pressure or must be discontinued because of the development of intolerable side effects.

Step 5—Creation of a Monitoring Plan

The pharmacist identifies specific monitoring parameters to assess the effectiveness of the regimen. The monitoring plan includes subjective and objective monitoring parameters for each drug in the therapeutic plan and is tailored to the practice site of the pharmacist. (Monitoring is discussed in detail in Chapter 8.) For example, community-based pharmacists rely more on subjective monitoring parameters than do institutional-based pharmacists, who have access to extensive objective patient data.

Step 6—Monitoring of the Patient and Modification of Regimens According to Patient Response

The clinical pharmacist must monitor the patient and adjust the therapeutic plan according to the patient's response to each medication in the therapeutic regimen. Several guidelines for altering the initial drug therapy are available (Box 7-5). If a specific therapeutic regimen appears ineffective, the pharmacist should ensure that the patient received an appropriate dose for an adequate amount of time and should question the patient closely about adherence to the prescribed or recommended regimen. Some drugs such as nonsteroidal antiinflammatory agents, cromolyn sodium, and antihypertensive agents require days to weeks of regular therapy before the maximal benefit of the drug is apparent. For drugs that have narrow therapeutic indexes, the pharmacist should ensure that the dosage is appropriate for the patient and the serum concentration is within the therapeutic range. For drugs that have wide therapeutic indexes, the pharmacist should maximize the dosage before deciding the agent is ineffective.

The patient's perception and ability to tolerate side effects may change with time. Some side effects may become more tolerable with time such as hand tremor with inhaled adrenergic agonists, headache with nitrates, and diuresis with hydrochlorothiazide, whereas other side effects are life threatening or intolerable to the patient such as anaphylaxis with penicillin, orthostatic hypotension with antihypertensives, and ulcerations of the gastric mucosa with nonsteroidal antiinflammatory drugs. The pharmacist must work to ensure that the patient understands the way to differentiate between mild and potentially serious side effects. Some side effects can be minimized by changing the time of day when the dose is taken such as taking diuretics in the morning rather than at bedtime to minimize nocturia or taking the dose with food such as taking theophylline with food to minimize stomach irritation. Other side effects can be minimized by adjusting the dosage of the drug. The pharmacist should avoid recommending the addition of other drugs to the patient's regimen simply for the purpose of counteracting the side effects of the original agent. Although additional agents are sometimes indicated, this process adds to the cost of therapy, increases the risk of drug interactions and additional side effects from the new agent, and unnecessarily complicates the therapeutic regimen, increasing the likelihood of noncompliance.

SUBJECTIVE OBJECTIVE ASSESSMENT PLAN FORMAT

The process of identifying the subjective and objective data, assessing the problem, and developing a specific therapeutic and monitoring plan is called SOAPing the problem. The term *SOAP* is an acronym for *Subjective Objective Assessment Plan*. The steps for SOAPing a problem include the following:
1. Creation of a list of related subjective parameters
2. Creation of a list of related objective parameters
3. Assessment and documentation of the problem
4. Documentation of the therapeutic plan for addressing the problem
The SOAP format provides a formal organizational structure.

Patient Case Example—Integration and Application

The steps involved in therapeutics planning (problem identification, problem prioritization, and selection of initial and alternate medication regimens) are illustrated in the following patient case.

Patient Case

Chief complaint: Referred to medicine clinic from orthopedic clinic for management of "high blood pressure" and asthma

History of present illness: CR is a 54-year-old African-American female who was referred to the medicine clinic for evaluation and management of her medical problems. She is being followed in the orthopedic clinic for a fracture of her left ankle, which occurred 2 weeks ago when she tripped over a curb. Her blood pressure at the time of the fracture was 150/100 mmHg. She also complained of a burning in her stomach that was relieved by eating or taking antacids. The burning often woke her at night; her upper gastrointestinal (UGI) series yesterday was significant for a duodenal ulcer. She has a 30-year history of asthma treated with daily prednisone. She complains of mild wheezing with exertion and when she breathes cold air.

Past medical history: Fractured left ankle, asthma for 30 years, status post (S/P) hernia repair age 18 years

Social history: Secretary; divorced mother of two; lives at home alone. Smoked one pack per day (ppd) for 3 years but quit 30 years ago. Social alcohol (drinks wine at parties or when dining out, three to four times per year for 30 years)

Review of systems: Weight gain despite numerous diets; moderate ankle pain

Medication History

Dietary: Has tried many weight-reduction diets in the past without success; currently not dieting

Allergies: Penicillin (was told she almost died as a child after being given a shot of penicillin)

Adverse drug reactions: Aspirin (causes wheezing)

Current prescription medications:

Prednisone 5 to 20 mg daily for "at least 20 years"

Acetaminophen with codeine (Tylenol No. 3) one to two tablets every 6 hours as needed for ankle pain; has taken at least two tablets daily for the past 2 weeks with good relief of pain for several hours after each dose

Past prescription medications: Has tried several different medications for her asthma but does not remember the names and cannot describe the medications. Does not remember using any prescription inhaled medications for her asthma

Current nonprescription medications:

Epinephrine (Bronkaid) metered dose inhaler (MDI) as needed (prn) for "years" (buys an inhaler every couple of weeks)

Antacids (Tums) one tablet prn indigestion; takes several doses per week off and on for "many years"

Past nonprescription medications: None that she can describe

Compliance: Appears to be compliant although says she has a hard time remembering to take her medications while at work. Decided on her own to take antacids. Does not see a physician regularly

Physical Examination

Pleasant, cooperative, obese female in no acute distress with a cast on her left ankle. Cushingoid facies and body habitus. 5'4", 185 lb

Vital Signs: Afebrile; blood pressure 148/105 mmHg; heart rate 75 beats per minute (BPM); respiratory rate 11 breaths per minute

Head eyes, ears, nose, and throat: Normocephalic and atraumatic (NCAT); extraocular muscles intact (EOMI); pupils equal, round, reactive to light and accommodation (PERRLA); tympanic membrane (TM) intact; oropharynx clear; copper wiring, AV nicking, and bilateral nasal polyps present

Cardiovascular: S_1, S_2, and S_4 present (distant heart sounds); point of maximal impulse (PMI) fifth intercostal space (5ICS) midclavicular line (MCL); no murmurs, rubs, or gallops

Lungs: Expiratory wheezing throughout all lung fields with slightly prolonged expiratory phase

Abdomen: Obese; normal active bowel sounds (NABS); tender right upper quadrant (RUQ); liver 12 cm; no spleen tip felt; abdominal scar

Extremities: No cyanosis, clubbing, or edema; pulses 2+ throughout; reflexes and strength within normal limits (WNL) upper extremities (UE) and lower extremities (LE) bilaterally (left lower extremity [LLE] not tested); cast on left ankle

Neurologic system: Nonfocal; cranial nerve (CN) II-XII intact

Laboratory Tests and Diagnostic Procedures

Chest x-ray (CXR) film (from emergency room [ER] 2 weeks ago): Clear with increased anteroposterior (AP) diameter

Electrocardiogram (ECG) (from ER 2 weeks ago): Sinus tachycardia

Panel 7 (from ER 2 weeks ago):

Sodium	140 mEq/L
Potassium	4.1 mEq/L
Chloride	110 mEq/L
Carbon dioxide content	25 mEq/L
Glucose	150 mg/dl
Creatinine	0.8 mg/dl

Complete blood count (CBC) (from ER 2 weeks ago):

White blood cells (WBC)	7200 cells/mm^3
Hemoglobin (Hgb)	12 g/dl
Hematocrit (HCT)	43%

Peak expiratory flow rate (PEFR): 320 L/min

Heme-positive stool

Duodenal ulcer on UGI series

Problem Identification

Step 1. Identification of subjective and objective patient parameters

Subjective parameters include the following:
- Burning stomach relieved by food and antacids
- Being awakened at night by burning in stomach
- Ankle pain requiring at least two Tylenol No. 3 daily
- Obesity despite trying numerous diets
- Wheezing with exertion and on breathing cold air
- History of "high blood pressure"
- History of asthma
- History of a surgical hernia repair
- History of penicillin allergy
- History of smoking
- History of aspirin intolerance

Objective parameters include the following:
- Fractured left ankle on x-ray film
- Prednisone 5 to 20 mg daily for "at least 20 years"
- Tylenol No. 3 one to two tablets every 6 hours prn ankle pain
- Epinephrine (Bronkaid) MDI prn for "years"
- Antacids (Tums) one tablet prn indigestion for "years"
- Blood pressure 148/105 mmHg
- 5'4", 185 lb
- Nasal polyps
- +S$_4$
- Distant heart sounds
- Obese abdomen
- Abdominal scar
- Expiratory wheezing

- Increased AP diameter
- PEFR 320 L/min
- Copper wiring
- AV nicking
- Heme-positive stool
- Duodenal ulcer on UGI series

Step 2. Creation of sets of related parameters. Possible groupings for parameters include the following:

1. Ankle group
   Subjective parameters: Ankle pain requiring at least two Tylenol No. 3 daily
   Objective parameters: Fractured left ankle on x-ray film; Tylenol No. 3 one to two tablets every 6 hours prn ankle pain
   Assessment: Fractured left ankle requiring prescription pain medication

2. Asthma group
   Subjective parameters: Wheezing with exertion and on breathing cold air; history of asthma
   Objective parameters: Expiratory wheezing; increased AP diameter; distant heart sounds; PEFR 320 L/min; prednisone 5 to 20 mg daily for "at least 20 years"; epinephrine (Bronkaid) MDI prn for "years"
   Assessment: Asthma symptomatic with exertion and exposure to cold air despite treatment with daily systemic corticosteroids and prn Bronkaid

3. Hypertension group
   Subjective parameters: History of "high blood pressure"
   Objective parameters: Blood pressure 148/105 mmHg; $+S_4$; copper wiring and AV nicking
   Assessment: Hypertension

4. Ulcer group
   Subjective parameters: Burning in stomach relieved by food and antacids; being awakened at night by burning in stomach
   Objective parameters: Antacids (Tums) one tablet prn indigestion for "years"; heme-positive stool; duodenal ulcer on UGI series
   Assessment: Duodenal ulcer

5. Penicillin allergy group
   Subjective parameters: History of a penicillin allergy
   Objective parameters: None
   Assessment: History of a penicillin allergy

6. Aspirin adverse reaction group
   Subjective parameters: History of aspirin intolerance; history of asthma
   Objective parameters: Nasal polyps
   Assessment: Aspirin intolerance

7. Hernia surgery group
   Subjective parameters: History of surgical hernia repair
   Objective parameters: Abdominal scar
   Assessment: S/P hernia repair

8. Obesity group
   Subjective parameters: Obesity despite numerous diets
   Objective parameters: 5'4", 185 lb
   Assessment: Obesity

9. Tobacco group
   Subjective parameters: Smoking history

Objective parameters: 3 pack-year smoking history

Assessment: Distant smoking history

Step 3. Creation of a patient problem list. The problem list (in no particular rank order) for the patient case is as follows:

1. Fractured left ankle
2. Asthma
3. Hypertension
4. Duodenal ulcer
5. History of penicillin allergy
6. History of aspirin intolerance
7. Obesity
8. S/P hernia repair
9. 3 pack-year smoking history

Problem Prioritization

Step 1. Identification of active patient problems. Active problems for the patient case include the following:

1. Fractured left ankle
2. Asthma
3. Hypertension
4. Duodenal ulcer
5. Obesity

Step 2. Identification of inactive patient problems. Inactive problems for the patient case include the following:

1. History of penicillin allergy
2. History of aspirin intolerance
3. S/P hernia repair
4. 3 pack-year smoking history

Step 3. Ranking of the problems. A prioritized list for the patient case follows:

Active problems requiring immediate therapeutic intervention include the following:

1. Duodenal ulcer
2. Hypertension
3. Asthma

Active problems requiring less immediate therapeutic intervention include the following:

4. Fractured left ankle (pain control)
5. Obesity

Inactive problems that require patient education but no therapeutic intervention include the following:

6. Aspirin intolerance
7. Penicillin allergy

Inactive problems that require no intervention include the following:

8. Smoking history
9. S/P hernia repair

The first three problems are of approximately equal importance in this patient, and their ranking is somewhat arbitrary. The fourth and fifth problems are active but can be addressed with less urgency than the first three problems. Problems six and seven do not require immediate therapeutic intervention but do require some patient intervention and may influence the choice of other medication regimens. Problems eight and nine are of historical interest only and require no therapeutic intervention.

Selection of Specific Therapeutic Regimens

Step 1. Creation of lists of all possible therapeutic options. The lists are as follows:

Problem 1—*Duodenal ulcer*

- Antacids (aluminum-containing products, magnesium-containing products, aluminum and magnesium combination products, sodium bicarbonate, calcium carbonate)
- *Helicobacter pylori* eradication regimens (single-agent bismuth or antibiotics, combination bismuth and antimicrobial regimens)
- H_2 receptor antagonists (cimetidine, famotidine, nizatidine, ranitidine)
- Prostaglandins (misoprostol)
- Proton-pump inhibitors (omeprazole, lansoprazole)
- Other (anticholinergics, cisapride, domperidone, metoclopramide, proglumide, somatostatin, zinc salts)

Problem 2—*Hypertension*

- Angiotensin-converting enzyme inhibitors (benazepril, captopril, enalapril, fosinopril, lisinopril, quinapril, ramipril)
- β-adrenergic receptor blockers (acebutolol, atenolol, betaxolol, carteolol, labetalol, nadolol, penbutolol, pindolol, propranolol, timolol)
- Calcium channel blockers (amlodipine, diltiazem, isradipine, nicardipine, nifedipine, felodipine, verapamil)
- Diuretics (potassium sparing, thiazides)
- Peripheral α_1-adrenergic receptor agonists (doxazosin, prazosin, terazosin)
- Peripheral α_1- and α_2-adrenergic receptor agonists (phentolamine, phenoxybenzamine)
- Postganglionic sympathetic inhibitors (guanadrel, guanethidine)
- Reserpine
- Vasodilators (hydralazine, minoxidil)

Problem 3—*Asthma*

- Short-acting adrenergic agonists (ephedrine, epinephrine, isoproterenol, isoetharine, bitolterol, metaproterenol, terbutaline, fenoterol, albuterol)
- Long-acting adrenergic agonists (salmeterol)
- Anticholinergics (atropine, ipratropium bromide)
- Aerosol corticosteroids (beclomethasone, budesonide flunisolide, fluticasone, triamcinolone)
- Systemic corticosteroids (betamethasone, dexamethasone, cortisone, hydrocortisone, methylprednisolone, prednisone, prednisolone, triamcinolone)
- Leukotriene modifiers (zafirlukast, zileuton)
- Mast cell stabilizers (cromolyn sodium, nedocromil sodium)
- Methylxanthines (aminophylline, theophylline)

Problem 4—*Fractured left ankle (pain control)*

- Acetic acids (etodolac, diclofenac)
- Acetaminophen
- Central nonnarcotics (tramadol)
- Morphine and morphine-like drugs (codeine, hydrocodone, hydromorphone, levorphanol, oxycodone, oxymorphone)
- Meperidine and meperidine-like drugs (fentanyl)
- Methadone and methadone-like drugs (propoxyphene)

- Mixed agonist-antagonists (buprenorphine, butorphanol, dezocine, nalbuphine, pentazocine)
- Propionic acids (ibuprofen, fenoprofen, ketoprofen, ketorolac, naproxen, naproxen sodium)
- Salicylates (aspirin, choline salicylate, diflunisal, magnesium salicylate, sodium salicylate)

Problem 5—*Obesity*

- Amphetamines (amphetamine, dextroamphetamine, methamphetamine)
- Nonamphetamines (benzphetamine, dexfenfluramine, diethylpropion, fenfluramine, mazindol, phendimetrazine, phenmetrazine, phentermine)
- Other (phenylpropanolamine)

Problem 6—*Aspirin intolerance:* No treatment options

Problem 7—*Penicillin allergy:* No treatment options

Problem 8—*Smoking history:* No treatment options

Problem 9—*S/P hernia repair:* No treatment options

Step 2. Elimination of therapeutic options based on the comparative effectiveness of the drugs, suitability of the drug for the patient, effectiveness of past treatment regimens, cost of therapy, formulary restrictions, and ability of the patient to comply with the proposed regimen.

Problem 1—*Duodenal ulcer:* The patient is an ambulatory patient who has trouble remembering to take her medication when at work. She needs a regimen that is simple, requires as few doses as possible, and is easily transportable. This is her first ulcer, so typical first-line regimens should be considered. She will have to take medications for her asthma and pain, so drug-drug interactions need to be considered. Systemic corticosteroids are ulcerogenic; chronic ulcer prophylaxis may be necessary depending on the regimen selected for the management of her asthma. Compliance with an appropriate antacid regimen (such as 30 ml of a highly potent antacid suspension 1 and 3 hours after meals and at bedtime for 4 to 6 weeks) may be difficult for this patient. Misoprostol is not indicated for the initial treatment of duodenal ulcers. Anticholinergics are less effective antagonists of acid secretion than H_2 receptor antagonists and should be used as adjuncts rather than as first-line agents. Therefore the following medications can be eliminated from consideration at this time: antacids, misoprostol, and anticholinergics.

Problem 2—*Hypertension:* The patient has never been treated for hypertension. Therefore typical first-line regimens should be considered. Race also is an important consideration. African-Americans commonly have a sodium- and volume-dependent hypertension responsive to diuretics or calcium channel blockers. In addition, the patient has asthma, which may be exacerbated by β-adrenergic blocking drugs, including the β_1-selective agents. Therefore the following medications can be eliminated from consideration at this time: angiotensin-converting enzyme inhibitors, β-adrenergic receptor blockers, central α_2-adrenergic receptor agonists, peripheral α_1- and α_2-adrenergic receptor agonists, postganglionic sympathetic inhibitors, reserpine, and vasodilators.

Problem 3—*Asthma:* The patient is on an unconventional asthma treatment regimen for her moderately severe asthma. She has apparently been self-treating with a short-acting nonselective nonprescription inhaled bronchodilator and has somehow had access to long-term oral corticosteroids. She is probably steroid dependent. Initial treatment of moderate asthma consists of scheduled inhaled antiinflammatory drugs (corticosteroids or mast cell stabilizers) and prn inhaled β_2-selective adrenergic agonists; additional bronchodilators may be added depending on patient response. Zafirlukast also is indicated for the prophylaxis and treatment of asthma. Mast cell stabilizers are less potent antiinflammatory drugs than are corticosteroids. Therefore the following medications can be eliminated from consideration at this time: ephedrine, epinephrine, isoproterenol, isoetharine, metaproterenol, salmeterol, atropine, ipratropium bromide, mast cell stabilizers, and methylxanthines.

Problem 4—*Fractured left ankle (pain control):* Pain is treated with the weakest effective analgesic with the fewest side effects. This patient appears to have relatively good pain control with her current acetaminophen and codeine regimen. Consideration of weaker analgesics is unreasonable. Conversely, parenteral drugs (narcotic and nonnarcotic) are not indicated for the management of mild to moderate pain in ambulatory patients. In addition, her aspirin-associated wheezing and the duodenal ulcer must be considered. All salicylates, salicylate-containing products, and nonsteroidal antiinflammatory agents (acetic acids, fenamates, and propionic acids) are contraindicated in patients with aspirin-associated wheezing. These same drugs irritate the gastrointestinal tract and should be avoided in this patient. Therefore the following drugs can be eliminated from consideration at this time: acetaminophen, aspirin, nonsteroidal antiinflammatory agents, parenteral opioid agonist-antagonists, and parenteral narcotics.

Problem 5—*Obesity:* Dietary intervention and exercise are considered first-line treatments for obesity; pharmacologic intervention is not indicated at this time. Therefore drug therapy is not considered at this time.

Problems 6, 7, 8, and 9: These problems do not require drug therapy.

Step 3. Selection of an appropriate therapeutic regimen, including drug, dosage, route, duration of therapy, and rationale.

Problem 1—*Duodenal ulcer:* Choices for the initial treatment of duodenal ulcer include combination regimens targeted at the eradication of *H. pylori,* H_2 receptor antagonists, and proton-pump inhibitors. Most duodenal ulcers are associated with *H. pylori* infection of the gastric mucosa. Definitive diagnosis requires invasive testing, and treatment is complex and inconvenient. The H_2 receptor antagonists, sucralfate, and proton inhibitors are equally effective in healing duodenal ulcers but do not eradicate *H. pylori.*

The following are two common treatment regimens for *H. pylori:*

1. A 2-week combination regimen consisting of metronidazole 500 mg three times a day (t.i.d.), tetracycline 500 mg four times a day (q.i.d.), bismuth subsalicylate two tablets q.i.d., and ranitidine 300 mg once daily followed by 4 more weeks of ranitidine
2. A 2-week combination regimen consisting of clarithromycin 500 mg t.i.d. and omeprazole (20 or 40 mg) once daily.

The second regimen is more convenient but costs about twice as much as the first regimen. Clarithromycin is associated with fewer adverse gastrointestinal side effects (nausea, vomiting, and diarrhea) than is metronidazole or tetracycline but may cause taste disturbances. Adverse effects associated with bismuth subsalicylate include a black tongue, black stools, and mild ringing of the ears. Bismuth subsalicylate contains salicylates and is therefore not indicated for this patient.

Regimens not targeted at eradication of *H. pylori* include 6 to 8 weeks of single daily doses of H_2 receptor antagonists, 6 to 8 weeks of multiple daily doses of sucralfate, or 4 weeks of single daily doses of a proton-pump inhibitor. H_2 receptor antagonists, sucralfate, and proton-pump inhibitors are associated with few side effects. However, H_2 receptor antagonists and proton-pump inhibitors interact with drugs such as theophylline that are metabolized by hepatic cytochrome P-450 enzymes.

Several equally effective regimens are available to treat this patient's duodenal ulcer. After consideration of all patient factors, one appropriate regimen is the 2-week combination regimen consisting of clarithromycin 500 mg t.i.d. and omeprazole 20 mg once daily.

Problem 2—*Hypertension:* Choices for the initial treatment of hypertension in this patient include diuretics and calcium channel blockers. In addition, contributing factors such as obesity and excessive salt intake should be minimized. Gradual weight reduction, exercise, and salt restriction to 6 grams per day or less minimizes factors contributing to her hypertension.

Diuretics and sustained-release dosage forms of calcium channel blockers can both be taken once daily. Diuretics and calcium channel blockers differ in cost and side effect profile. Diuretics are less expensive than are calcium channel blockers. Diuretic-associated side effects include hypokalemia, hypomagnesemia, hypercalcemia, hyperuricemia, hyperlipidemia, and sexual dysfunction. Patients usually require potassium supplementation for diuretic-associated hypokalemia. All calcium channel blockers may cause gastrointestinal disturbances. Other calcium channel blocker associated side effects are drug specific. Diltiazem and verapamil may decrease heart rate, slow AV conduction, and cause heart failure in patients with borderline cardiac reserve. Nifedipine may cause dizziness, flushing, headache, peripheral edema, and mood changes.

Diuretics are generally considered the initial drugs of choice for this type of patient. Of the four classes of diuretics (thiazides, thiazide-like, loops, and carbonic anhydrase inhibitors), the thiazide diuretics are the most effective drugs if patients have adequate renal function; this patient has an estimated creatinine clearance of approximately 70 ml/min. All thiazides and thiazide-like diuretics are equally effective. Low doses (12.5 to 25 mg of hydrochlorothiazide and 25 mg of chlorthalidone) minimize electrolyte loss.

Several equally appropriate regimens are available to treat hypertension in this patient. After consideration of all patient factors, one appropriate regimen is hydrochlorothiazide 12.5 mg daily, weight reduction, exercise, and salt restriction.

Problem 3—*Asthma:* This patient should be started on scheduled inhaled corticosteroids and prn inhaled β_2-adrenergic agonists; the prednisone should be tapered slowly over several months as tolerated. No clinical difference exists among the inhaled corticosteroids (beclomethasone, budesonide, triamcinolone, flunisolide, and fluticasone). All five may be administered twice daily. All five may cause oral candidiasis and dysphonia; these side effects may be minimized by administering the drug with a spacer device and rinsing the mouth and gargling after each dose. Beclomethasone is an older product and therefore may be less expensive. Zafirlukast is administered orally twice daily and is associated with few side effects. No clinical difference exists among the four available inhaled β_2-adrenergic agonists (albuterol, fenoterol, pirbuterol, and terbutaline); albuterol is the most commonly prescribed agent. Side effects with all four drugs include hand tremor and tachycardia. All four drugs are administered in a dose of one to two puffs every 4 to 6 hours as needed.

Several equally efficacious regimens are available to treat asthma in this patient. After consideration of all patient factors, an appropriate regimen is beclomethasone four puffs twice daily, prednisone taper (decrease the daily dose by 2.5 mg weekly as tolerated), and albuterol one to two puffs every 4 to 6 hours as needed.

Problem 4—*Fractured ankle (pain control):* The patient appears to be doing well on her current regimen of one to two tablets of Tylenol No. 3 (acetaminophen 300 mg with codeine 30 mg) every 6 hours prn pain. The regimen is appropriate for the patient and does not need to be changed.

Problem 5—*Obesity:* Pharmacologic therapy is not indicated at this time.

Problem 6—*Aspirin intolerance:* Pharmacologic therapy is not indicated. However, the patient should be counseled about avoiding aspirin-containing products and nonsteroidal antiinflammatory agents. Many nonprescription products contain aspirin and other salicylates. The patient should be provided with a list of products containing these ingredients and advised to check with her pharmacist or physician before purchasing any nonprescription product.

Problems 7, 8, and 9: No therapeutic interventions required

Step 4. Identification of alternate therapeutic regimens

Problem 1—*Duodenal ulcer:* A second course of *H. pylori* treatment should be considered if the ulcer does not heal or symptoms recur. Poor compliance and microbial resistance should be considered if the ulcer does not heal with a second course of treatment. Long-term, low-dosage therapy with an H_2 blocker, proton-pump inhibitor, or sucralfate should be considered if the patient relapses within 3 to 6 months or has two or more ulcers during a 12-month period.

Problem 2—*Hypertension:* The dose of the thiazide diuretic can be increased to 25 mg daily if blood pressure is not controlled with the initial regimen. Check for patient adherence to the recommended drug therapy, dietary restrictions, and exercise program. A calcium channel blocker can be substituted for the thiazide diuretic if the blood pressure remains inadequately controlled. The combination of a diuretic and calcium channel blocker is effective for the management of low-renin, volume-expanded hypertension and can be considered if monotherapy is ineffective. If the patient experiences intolerable side effects while taking a calcium channel antagonist, the pharmacist should consider changing drugs within the class. The pharmacist should change classes of drugs if the side effect is common to all drugs within the class.

Problem 3—*Asthma:* The dose of the inhaled corticosteroid can be increased and the prednisone taper delayed or slowed if the patient experiences more symptoms as the systemic dose is reduced. Zafirlukast may be added in place of the inhaled corticosteroid. A long-acting bronchodilator (salmeterol or sustained-release theophylline) can be added to the regimen.

Problem 4—*Fractured ankle (pain control):* The dosage and frequency of Tylenol No. 3 can be changed if the patient has inadequate pain control on the current regimen. Constipation is a common patient complaint with codeine-containing regimens and can be addressed by adding a stool softener and a high-fiber diet.

Problem 5—*Obesity:* A variety of dietary and exercise programs are available. Some patients benefit from weekly support group meetings; other patients prefer more one-on-one support. Anorexiants can be considered as adjuncts if the patient fails a reasonable diet and exercise program. Sympathomimetics (phentermine, phenylpropanolamine) should be avoided in patients with hypertension. Dexfenfluramine or fenfluramine may be used as an adjunct to diet and exercise.

Problems 6, 7, 8, and 9: No drug treatment required. No alternative treatment regimens necessary.

Initial Treatment Regimen

Consideration of all patient problems and therapeutic issues results in the following initial treatment regimen:

- Clarithyromycin 500 mg t.i.d. for 2 weeks
- Omeprazole 20 mg once daily for 2 weeks
- Hydrochlorothiazide 12.5 mg daily
- Beclomethasone four puffs twice daily
- Prednisone taper (decrease the daily dose by 2.5 mg weekly as tolerated)
- Albuterol one to two puffs every 4 to 6 hours as needed
- Acetaminophen 300 mg with codeine 30 mg one to two tablets every 6 hours prn pain
- Weight reduction and exercise program
- Salt restriction to 6 grams per day or less

SELF-ASSESSMENT QUESTIONS

1 Which one of the following is NOT a component of the planning process?
   a. Problem identification
   b. Problem prioritization
   c. Selection of specific initial and alternative treatment regimens
   d. Development of an integrated monitoring plan
   e. Patient counseling

2 Which one of the following is NOT a step involved in the identification of patient problems?
   a. Identification of subjective and objective patient parameters
   b. Creation of a working list of all patient parameters
   c. Prioritization of patient parameters
   d. Creation of sets of related problems
   e. Determination of each specific patient problem

3 Which one of the following is a subjective parameter?
   a. Serum creatinine
   b. Weight
   c. Height
   d. Dysuria
   e. Peak expiratory flow rate

4 Which one of the following is NOT a subjective parameter?
   a. Anxiety
   b. Indigestion

    c. Respiratory rate
    d. Insomnia
    e. Pain

5 Which one of the following is an objective parameter?
    a. Blurred vision
    b. Temperature
    c. Headache
    d. Tinnitus
    e. Fatigue

6 Which one of the following is NOT an objective parameter?
    a. Vertigo
    b. Urine output
    c. Bilirubin
    d. Hemoglobin
    e. Ejection fraction

7 A patient arrives in the emergency room with a serious head injury. Laboratory tests identify mild hyperlipidemia. The patient is S/P a hernia repair. Which of the following is an appropriate prioritization of the patient's problems?

PROBLEM #1	PROBLEM #2	PROBLEM #3
a. Head injury	Hyperlipidemia	S/P hernia repair
b. S/P hernia repair	Hyperlipidemia	Head injury
c. Hyperlipidemia	S/P hernia repair	Head injury
d. Hyperlipidemia	Head injury	S/P hernia repair
e. Head injury	S/P hernia repair	Hyperlipidemia

8 A patient arrives at the medication refill clinic requesting a refill of her antihypertensive medication. She states that "It is hard to get around because my feet have been so swollen." Physical examination reveals bilateral 4+ pitting edema to the knees, scattered crackles in all lung fields, jugular venous distention, and a displaced point of maximal impulse. Blood pressure is 120/78 mmHg. She has a penicillin allergy. Which of the following is an appropriate prioritization of the patient's problems?

PROBLEM #1	PROBLEM #2	PROBLEM #3
a. Hypertension	Penicillin allergy	Congestive heart failure
b. Hypertension	Congestive heart failure	Penicillin allergy
c. Congestive heart failure	Hypertension	Penicillin allergy
d. Congestive heart failure	Penicillin allergy	Hypertension
e. Penicillin allergy	Congestive heart failure	Hypertension

9 Which of the following is NOT a step in the selection of specific therapeutic regimens?
    a. Creation of a list of therapeutic options for each problem
    b. Selection of an appropriate therapeutic regimen for each problem
    c. Identification of alternative regimens
    d. Creation of a monitoring plan and monitoring of the patient
    e. Identification of objective and subjective patient parameters

10 A patient with a dry, hacking cough asks the pharmacist to recommend a cough medication. The pharmacist, who does not know the patient, recommends a popular nonprescription cough suppressant without checking the patient's medication profile. What error did the pharmacist commit?

a. The pharmacist should have considered other patient problems.
b. The pharmacist should have recommended an expectorant.
c. The pharmacist should have advised the patient to see a physician.
d. The pharmacist should have recommended a decongestant.
e. The pharmacist should have obtained a prescription for a cough suppressant from the patient's doctor.

C H A P T E R 8

Monitoring Drug Therapies

LEARNING OBJECTIVES

1 Identify the skills needed to monitor patients.
2 List and describe each step in the monitoring process.
3 Identify the four types of monitoring data included in the four-square monitoring method.
4 Given specific monitoring parameters, organize patient data appropriately.

MONITORING drug therapy provides the information necessary to determine whether the therapeutic regimen is achieving the expected or desired outcome or needs to be changed because of lack of response or the development of undesirable or potentially dangerous adverse drug reactions. Most pharmacists spend a significant amount of their time monitoring patient response to drug therapy. Recommended interventions based on monitoring results are verbally communicated directly to the health care team or documented in the patient medical record.

Pharmacists need a variety of skills to assess patient-specific monitoring parameters and the appropriateness of therapeutic regimens. Pharmacists must have an excellent knowledge of pharmacotherapeutics and pathophysiology and understand the application and interpretation of a wide variety of laboratory and diagnostic tests. Although results of laboratory and diagnostic tests have traditionally been accessible only in inpatient settings, access to this type of data is increasing in the ambulatory care setting. Other important skills include communication and physical assessment skills.

A great deal of information about response to therapy and the presence of undesirable or potentially dangerous adverse drug reactions can be obtained by questioning patients regarding their experiences, both positive and negative, with their medications. Simple physical examination assessment parameters such as blood pressure and heart and respiratory rate may be useful in monitoring the response to many therapeutic regimens. More comprehensive physical assessment skills may be needed for monitoring more complex therapeutic regimens.

The amount of subjective and objective data obtained from and about a patient may be extensive. For example, results from 10 or more laboratory tests may be available several times a day for patients in the critical care inpatient setting. Therefore in addition to having an excellent knowledge of pharmacotherapeutics, pathophysiology, laboratory and diagnostic tests, and physical assessment parameters, the pharmacist needs a structured, ordered process for the selection, organization, documentation, and assessment of subjective and objective data. This chapter introduces a structured process and approach to monitoring drug therapy.

PROCESS

Monitoring is an organized and dynamic process (Box 8-1). The initial drug monitoring plan should be developed at the time the initial therapeutic plan is created and then adjusted according to patient response and changes in the therapeutic regimen.

Step 1—Set Therapeutic Goals

The specific goals and outcomes of therapy should be determined before any other planning takes place. Specific goals should be set for each patient problem and for the therapeutic outcome in general. Target ranges for all objective parameters (such as serum potassium between 3.5 and 4.5 mEq/L) and target subjective responses for all subjective parameters (such as the ability to sleep through the night without wheezing) should be identified. The pharmacist also must consider long-term goals such as the impact of the therapeutic regimen on the patient's quality of life and survival.

Factors to consider when setting goals of therapy include the severity of disease and the acuity or chronicity of therapy. For example, the pharmacist should consider the differences in the goals of insulin therapy for a young patient with newly diagnosed insulin-dependent diabetes mellitus and an elderly patient with a 50-year history of insulin-dependent diabetes mellitus and significant cardiovascular and peripheral vascular disease. Because evidence suggests that tight control of blood sugar levels may delay the onset of the complications of diabetes and decrease their severity after they occur, the target blood sugar level for the young, newly diagnosed patient with diabetes may be lower and narrower than it is for the elderly patient with diabetes and long-standing disease who has already developed complications from the disease and is at risk from hypoglycemic episodes. Another example is the difference in the goals of antihypertensive therapy for a patient with a hypertensive emergency and signs of end-organ damage and a patient with newly diagnosed mild-to-moderate hypertension. The goal of therapy for the patient with malignant hypertension is to lower but not normalize the blood pressure quickly; this may require the use of parenteral antihypertensive agents and nearly minute-to-minute assessment of the patient's response to therapy. The goal of therapy for the patient with newly diagnosed mild-to-moderate hypertension is a blood pressure of approximately 125/85 mmHg. Drug therapy should be initiated, but the goal may not be reached for several weeks; the patient's response to therapy is assessed every 1 to 2 weeks.

Box 8-1	*The Process of Monitoring Therapeutic Regimens*

Step 1	Set therapeutic goals.
Step 2	Determine specific monitoring parameters.
Step 3	Integrate the monitoring plan.
Step 4	Monitor the patient's response to therapy.
Step 5	Assess the response to therapy.
Step 6	Alter the therapeutic regimen if necessary.
Step 7	Repeat Steps 1 to 6.

Step 2—Determine Specific Monitoring Parameters

Two possible outcomes exist for all medication regimens:

1. The medication regimen provides the expected therapeutic benefit for the patient.
2. The medication regimen does not provide the expected therapeutic benefit or is otherwise harmful to the patient.

These two outcomes can be assessed by monitoring patient-specific subjective and objective data. (See Boxes 7-2 and 7-3 on page 139 for examples of subjective and objective data.)

Subjective and objective data can be obtained for each of the two therapeutic outcomes, resulting in four distinct sets of monitoring data available to the clinical pharmacist.

1. *Subjective-Therapeutic*—Subjective data for assessing whether the medication regimen provides the expected therapeutic outcome
2. *Subjective-Toxic*—Subjective data for assessing whether the medication regimen does not provide the expected therapeutic outcome or is otherwise harmful to the patient
3. *Objective-Therapeutic*—Objective data for assessing whether the medication regimen provides the expected therapeutic outcome
4. *Objective-Toxic*—Objective data for assessing whether the medication regimen does not provide the expected therapeutic outcome or is otherwise harmful to the patient

These four sets of monitoring data may be organized using a visual process such as four subdivisions of a large square (the four-square method) (Figure 8-1). Each subdivision of the larger square represents one of the four sets of monitoring data described previously (subjective-therapeutic, subjective-toxic, objective-therapeutic, objective-toxic). The large square represents the monitoring plan for each medication.

Monitoring parameters are selected for each type of data and listed in the appropriate subdivision of the large square. The process is repeated for each medication in the therapeutic regimen, providing the pharmacist with a monitoring plan for each medication. This approach not only provides the pharmacist with an organized and thorough monitoring plan but also reminds the pharmacist of the relationships among the types of monitoring data and the reasons for evaluating any specific parameter.

In selecting specific subjective and objective monitoring parameters, the pharmacist should consider the pharmacotherapeutics and indications of each medication in the regimen. If the medication provides the expected therapeutic outcome, patient symptoms should decrease or disappear. Therefore as a first step the pharmacist should identify current patient symptoms. The pharmacist also should identify any abnormal objective findings such as elevated blood pressure, decreased peak flow rate, increased weight, decreased ejection fraction, and subtherapeutic serum drug concentration. These abnormal objective parameters should return to normal or at least to acceptable values if the medication produces the expected therapeutic outcome. The pharmacist also should consider the potential adverse effects attributed to the specific medication and identify patient complaints and objective parameters that may help identify adverse effects. For example, theophylline may cause nausea and cardiac stimulation. A patient can describe the nausea; checking the heart rate may confirm tachycardia.

Subjective—Therapeutic	Subjective—Toxic
Objective—Therapeutic	Objective—Toxic

FIGURE 8-1 *Organization of Monitoring Parameters (The Four-Square Method).* *Subjective-therapeutic* monitoring parameters are subjective data for the expected therapeutic outcome. *Subjective-toxic* monitoring parameters are subjective data indicating therapeutic failure or harm to the patient. *Objective-therapeutic* monitoring parameters are objective data for the expected therapeutic outcome. *Objective-toxic* monitoring parameters are objective data indicating therapeutic failure or harm to the patient.

Step 3—Integrate the Monitoring Plan

No integration is required if the patient is receiving just one medication. However, most patients receive multiple drugs; therefore the individual medication monitoring plans must be integrated into one master monitoring plan. One way to integrate the monitoring plan is to create a master list of subjective and objective monitoring parameters collated from each of the individual medication monitoring plans, noting all the reasons for monitoring any given parameter. For example, heart rate may be an objective monitoring parameter for the therapeutic and toxic response to digoxin, the therapeutic response to furosemide, and the toxic response to theophylline. To monitor the heart rate, the pharmacist needs only to measure or look up the heart rate response; however, the pharmacist must consider all the reasons for monitoring heart rate when assessing the actual response.

Step 4—Monitor the Patient's Response to Therapy

After the monitoring plan has been developed, the pharmacist begins monitoring the patient's response to therapy. The pharmacist can obtain responses for subjective monitoring parameters by interviewing the patient or caregiver. Objective monitoring data can be obtained from the patient medical record or computerized laboratory reporting systems.

The frequency of monitoring depends on the acuteness and severity of the illness and the risks associated with the specific drug therapy. For example, patients receiving experimental combination drug therapy for the treatment of cancer need to be monitored more acutely and frequently than do patients receiving daily aspirin therapy for the prevention of cardiovascular disease. Ambulatory patients with relatively stable disease may need to be monitored as infrequently as every few months, whereas critically ill patients may need to be monitored continuously.

The data obtained must be documented in an organized, easily accessible format. In general, subjective and objective responses should be documented separately. Flow sheets work well for documenting objective data; brief sequential serial notes work well for documenting subjective data. Most pharmacists prefer to create their own customized monitoring forms that provide a structured format for the organization of practice-specific data. Some pharmacists use institution-specific monitoring forms that have been developed and agreed on by consensus. Figures 8-2 and 8-3 are examples of medication flow sheets and Figures 8-4 through 8-6 are examples of objective data flow sheets.

Step 5—Assess the Response to Therapy

The pharmacist continuously evaluates the patient's response to therapy by assessing the subjective and objective monitoring parameters. The identification of trends is as important as the identification of single, marked changes. For example, a single hypoglycemic reaction to a larger-than-necessary dose of insulin is as important as a slowly decreasing serum platelet count. No changes should be made to the therapeutic regimen if the response is appropriate. However, the therapeutic regimen should be modified if it does not achieve the desired therapeutic outcome or is associated with intolerable or potentially dangerous adverse effects.

Step 6—Alter the Therapeutic Regimen if Necessary

Changes in the therapeutic regimen are made as indicated by the response to the regimen. Dosages may be increased or decreased; drugs may be deleted or added to the regimen. All changes are made according to the therapeutic plan, and a modified or new monitoring plan is developed.

Text continued on p. 168

Start Date	Stop Date	Medication, Dose, Route, Schedule									

FIGURE 8-2 *Flow Sheet for Scheduled Medications.* Example of a flow sheet for monitoring scheduled medications.

Start Date	Stop Date	Medication, Dose, Route, Schedule	Doses Given									

FIGURE 8-3 *Flow Sheet for "As Needed" (prn) Medications.* Example of a flow sheet for monitoring prn medications.

Date
Chemistry
Na
K
Cl
CO_2
Glucose
BUN
Creatinine
Calcium
Phosphorus
Uric acid
Bilirubin—total
Bilirubin—direct
Protein—total
Albumin
Globulin
LDH
AST
ALT
CPK
AP
Amylase
NH_3
Other

Hematology													
Hgb													
HCT													
WBC													
Polymorphonuclear leukocytes													
Bands													
Lymphocytes													
Eosinophils													
Monocytes													
Basophils													
Atypical lymphocytes													
Other													
Erythrocyte sedimentation rate													
Reticulocytes													
Platelets													
PT/PTT													
Blood Gases													
FIO_2													
pH													
PCO_2													
PO_2													
HCO_3													
% Saturation													
P (A-a) O_2													

FIGURE 8-4 *Laboratory Flow Sheet.* Example of a flow sheet for monitoring laboratory data.

Date												
BP												
HR												
CO												
CI												
CVP												
MAP												
PAP												
PCWP												
RAP												
PVR												
SvR												
CaO_2												
CVO_2												

FIGURE 8-5 *Hemodynamics Flow Sheet.* Example of a flow sheet for monitoring hemodynamic data.

Date	Site	Gram's Stain	Organism	Susceptibilities	
				Sensitive	Resistant

FIGURE 8-6 *Microbiology Flow Sheet.* Example of a flow sheet for monitoring microbiology data.

APPLICATION AND INTEGRATION

The following example illustrates the steps in the monitoring process.

Case Study

JC, a 69-year-old white male with a diagnosis of right- and left-sided congestive heart failure, complains of swollen feet, shortness of breath when walking more than half a block, nonproductive cough that is worse at night, and occasional leg cramps. He gained 30 lb over the past 3 months and notes that all his clothes are too tight. He props himself up with three pillows when sleeping. The goal of therapy is to improve the patient's quality of life by improving cardiac function and controlling symptoms. His new medication regimen includes digoxin (Lanoxin) 0.25 mg daily, furosemide (Lasix) 40 mg daily, captopril (Capoten) 25 mg three times daily, and potassium chloride (Slow-K) 8 mEq three times daily.

Digoxin Monitoring Parameters (Figure 8-7)

Subjective-Therapeutic Monitoring Parameters—The patient's symptoms should diminish or disappear if digoxin therapy provides the expected therapeutic benefit of improved cardiac function. Subjective-therapeutic monitoring parameters for digoxin include the following: decreased swelling of the feet, looser-fitting clothing, decreased shortness of breath with exertion, increased exercise tolerance, the ability to sleep lying down or with fewer pillows, and decreased cough.

Subjective-Toxic Monitoring Parameters—The patient's symptoms will not improve and may worsen if digoxin therapy does not provide the expected therapeutic benefit; the patient also may experience a variety of annoying or potentially harmful side effects from digoxin therapy. Subjective-toxic monitoring parameters for digoxin include the following: increased swelling of the feet, tighter-fitting clothing, increased shortness of breath with exertion, decreased exercise tolerance, more problems sleeping, increased cough, decreased appetite or loss of appetite, nausea, vomiting, visual disturbances such as halos around lights or yellowish visual tinting, abdominal discomfort, palpitations, weakness, lethargy, and agitation or disorientation.

Objective-Therapeutic Monitoring Parameters—A variety of laboratory and other tests are used to monitor improvement in cardiac function from digoxin therapy. Improvement in cardiac function may not be immediately evident after initiation of treatment but may be identified with long-term drug therapy. Objective-therapeutic monitoring parameters include the following: decreased edema and heart size on chest x-ray films; decreased weight; increased ejection fraction; and improved R wave progression V_1 to V_6, normalization of the S to R relationship, and decreased T wave inversion and asymmetry on electrocardiogram (ECG).

Objective-Toxic Monitoring Parameters—A variety of laboratory and other tests are used to monitor for lack of improvement in cardiac function or potentially harmful side effects from digoxin therapy. Objective-toxic monitoring parameters for digoxin include the following: increased edema and heart size on chest x-ray films; increased weight; decreased ejection fraction; poor R wave progression V_1 to V_6, abnormal S to R relationship, increased T wave inversion and asymmetry, and premature ventricular contractions on ECG; arrhythmias (bigeminy, trigeminy, ventricular tachycardia, ventricular fibrillation, atrial fibril-

Subjective—Therapeutic	Subjective—Toxic
↓ Swelling of feet Looser-fitting clothing ↓ SOB and DOE ↑ Exercise tolerance Sleeps with fewer pillows ↓ Cough	↑ Swelling of feet Tighter-fitting clothing ↑ SOB and DOE ↓ Exercise tolerance More problems sleeping ↑ Cough ↓ Or loss of appetite Nausea Vomiting Halos around lights Yellowish visual tinting Abdominal discomfort Palpitations Weakness Lethargy Agitation or disorientation
Objective—Therapeutic	Objective—Toxic
↓ Heart size on CXR ↓ Edema on CXR ↓ Weight ↑ Ejection fraction Improved R wave progression Normalization of S:R ↓ T wave inversion	↑ Heart size on CXR ↑ Edema on CXR ↑ Weight ↓ Ejection fraction Poor R wave progression Abnormal S:R ↑ T wave inversion VPDs Cardiac arrhythmias Serum digoxin greater than 2 ng/ml ↓ Heart rate ↓ Blood pressure

FIGURE 8-7 *Digoxin Monitoring Plan.* Example of subjective and objective monitoring parameters for digoxin.

lation); serum digoxin concentration greater than 2 ng/ml; decreased heart rate; and decreased blood pressure.

Furosemide Monitoring Parameters (Figure 8-8)

Subjective-Therapeutic Monitoring Parameters—The patient's symptoms should decrease or disappear if furosemide therapy provides the expected therapeutic benefit of improving cardiac function by decreasing intravascular volume. Subjective-therapeutic monitoring parameters for furosemide include the following: decreased swelling of the feet, looser-fitting clothing, decreased shortness of breath with exertion, increased exercise tolerance, ability to sleep lying down or with fewer pillows, and decreased cough.

Subjective—Therapeutic	Subjective—Toxic
↓ Swelling of feet Looser-fitting clothing ↓ SOB and DOE Able to sleep with fewer pillows ↓ Cough	↑ Swelling of feet Tighter-fitting clothing ↑ SOB and DOE More problems sleeping ↑ Cough Muscle cramps Dry mouth Thirst Dizziness Upset stomach Weakness Palpitations Lethargy Confusion
Objective—Therapeutic	Objective—Toxic
↓ Heart size on CXR ↓ Edema on CXR ↓ Weight ↑ Ejection fraction Improved R wave progression Normalization of S:R ↓ T wave inversion	↑ Heart size on CXR ↑ Edema on CXR ↑ Weight ↓ Ejection fraction Poor R wave progression Abnormal S:R ↑ T wave inversion ↓ Serum potassium ↑ Serum glucose ↑ Serum uric acid ↑ Serum BUN/serum creatinine ratio ↑ Serum BUN ↑ Serum creatinine ↓ Blood pressure ↑ Heart rate U wave or flat or inverted T wave

FIGURE 8-8 *Furosemide Monitoring Plan.* Example of subjective and objective monitoring parameters for furosemide.

Subjective-Toxic Monitoring Parameters—The patient's symptoms will not improve and may worsen if furosemide therapy does not provide the expected therapeutic benefit. The patient also may experience a variety of annoying or potentially harmful side effects from furosemide therapy. Subjective-toxic monitoring parameters for furosemide include the following: increased swelling of the feet, tighter-fitting clothing, increased shortness of breath with exertion, decreased exercise tolerance, more problems sleeping, increased cough, muscle cramps, dry mouth, thirst, dizziness (especially on arising from bed or standing), upset stomach, weakness, palpitations, lethargy, and confusion.

Objective-Therapeutic Monitoring Parameters—A variety of laboratory and other tests are used to monitor improvement in the fluid overload status of the patient. Some improvement in cardiac function may occur as a result of diuretic therapy. Objective-therapeutic monitoring parameters include the following: decreased edema and heart size on chest x-ray films; decreased weight; increased ejection fraction; and improved R wave progression V_1 to V_6, normalization of the S to R relationship, and decreased T wave inversion and asymmetry on ECG.

Objective-Toxic Monitoring Parameters—A variety of laboratory and other tests are used to monitor for lack of improvement in cardiac function or potentially harmful side effects from furosemide therapy. Objective-toxic monitoring parameters for furosemide include the following: increased edema and heart size on chest x-ray films; increased weight; decreased ejection fraction; poor R wave progression V_1 to V_6, abnormal S to R relationship, U wave or flat or inverted T wave, and increased T wave inversion and asymmetry on ECG; decreased serum potassium; increased serum glucose; increased serum uric acid; increased serum blood urea nitrogen to serum creatinine ratio; increased serum blood urea nitrogen; increased serum creatinine; decreased blood pressure; and increased heart rate.

Captopril Monitoring Parameters (Figure 8-9)

Subjective-Therapeutic Monitoring Parameters—If captopril therapy provides the expected therapeutic benefit of improved cardiac function, the patient's symptoms should decrease or disappear. Subjective-therapeutic monitoring parameters for captopril include the following: decreased swelling of the feet, looser-fitting clothing, decreased shortness of breath with exertion, increased exercise tolerance, ability to sleep lying down or with fewer pillows, and decreased cough.

Subjective-Toxic Monitoring Parameters—If captopril therapy does not provide the expected therapeutic benefit, the patient's symptoms will not improve and may worsen. The patient also may experience a variety of annoying or potentially harmful side effects from captopril therapy. Subjective-toxic monitoring parameters for captopril include the following: increased swelling of the feet, tighter-fitting clothing, increased shortness of breath with exertion, decreased exercise tolerance, more problems sleeping, persistent dry cough, dizziness (especially on arising or standing), itching, maculopapular or morbilliform rash, and dysgeusia.

Objective-Therapeutic Monitoring Parameters—A variety of laboratory and other tests are used to monitor improvement in cardiac function. Improvement in cardiac function may not be immediately evident after initiation of treatment but may be noted after long-term drug administration. Objective-therapeutic monitoring parameters for captopril include the following: decreased edema and heart size on chest x-ray films; decreased weight; increased ejection fraction; and improved R wave progression V_1 to V_6, normalization of the S to R relationship, and decreased T wave inversion and asymmetry on ECG.

Objective-Toxic Monitoring Parameters—A variety of laboratory and other tests are used to monitor for lack of improvement in cardiac function or potentially harmful side effects from captopril therapy. Objective-toxic monitoring parameters for captopril include the following: increased edema and heart size on chest x-ray films; increased weight; decreased ejection fraction; poor R wave progression V_1 to V_6, abnormal S to R relationship, and increased T

Subjective—Therapeutic ↓ Swelling of feet Looser-fitting clothes ↓ SOB and DOE ↑ Exercise tolerance Able to sleep with fewer pillows ↓ Cough	Subjective—Toxic ↑ Swelling of feet Tighter-fitting clothes ↑ SOB and DOE ↓ Exercise tolerance More problems sleeping Persistent dry cough Dizziness Itching Maculopapular or morbilliform rash Dysgeusia
Objective—Therapeutic ↓ Heart size on CXR ↓ Edema on CXR ↓ Weight ↑ Ejection fraction Improved R wave progression Normalization of S:R ↓ T wave inversion	Objective—Toxic ↑ Heart size on CXR ↑ Edema on CXR ↑ Weight ↓ Ejection fraction Poor R wave progression Abnormal S:R ↑ T wave inversion Elevated temperature Eosinophilia Proteinuria ↑ Serum creatinine ↑ Serum BUN ↓ Blood pressure WBC with differential

FIGURE 8-9 *Captopril Monitoring Plan.* Example of subjective and objective monitoring parameters for captopril.

wave inversion and asymmetry on ECG; elevated temperature; eosinophilia; proteinuria; increased serum creatinine; increased serum blood urea nitrogen; decreased blood pressure; and abnormal white blood cell count with differential.

Potassium Chloride Monitoring Parameters (Figure 8-10)

Subjective-Therapeutic Monitoring Parameters—The patient is receiving supplemental potassium to prevent hypokalemia resulting from the furosemide therapy. Because this is preventive therapy, no subjective parameters are available to evaluate the desired outcome of supplemental potassium therapy.

Subjective-Toxic Monitoring Parameters—The patient may develop hypokalemia if potassium supplementation is inadequate. Conversely, if potassium supplementation is excessive, the patient may experience symptoms of hyperkalemia. Subjective-toxic monitoring parameters for potassium chloride include the fol-

Subjective—Therapeutic	Subjective—Toxic
	Nausea
	Vomiting
	Diarrhea
	Bad taste
	Abdominal discomfort
	Palpitations
	Lethargy
	Weakness
	Muscle cramps
Objective—Therapeutic	**Objective—Toxic**
Serum potassium	Serum potassium
	Flattened P wave
	Widened QRS complex
	Peaked T wave
	Flattened or inverted T waves
	U waves

FIGURE 8-10 *Potassium Chloride Monitoring Plan.* Example of subjective and objective monitoring parameters for potassium chloride.

lowing: nausea, vomiting, diarrhea, bad taste, abdominal discomfort, palpitations, lethargy, weakness, and muscle cramps.

Objective-Therapeutic Monitoring Parameters—The goal of therapy is to maintain an appropriate serum potassium level with supplemental therapy. Objective-therapeutic monitoring parameters include serum potassium levels.

Objective-Toxic Monitoring Parameters—Objective monitoring parameters for supplemental potassium therapy are limited and include the following: serum potassium levels and flattened P wave, widened QRS complex, and peaked T wave on ECG (hyperkalemia) and flattened or inverted T wave and U wave on ECG (hypokalemia).

Integrated Monitoring Plan (Figures 8-11 and 8-12)

All the drugs in the therapeutic regimen are prescribed for the management of congestive heart failure. Therefore a great deal of duplication occurs among the monitoring plans. However, the pharmacist must go through this cognitive process to identify the many reasons for monitoring any given parameter. The patient should be monitored daily for initial response to therapy, and then less frequently as the patient's condition stabilizes. Therapeutic monitoring is an ongoing process, with modifications in the regimen and monitoring plan made according to the patient's response to therapy.

Subjective—Therapeutic	Subjective—Toxic
↓ Swelling of feet Looser-fitting clothes ↓ SOB and DOE ↑ Exercise tolerance Able to sleep with fewer pillows ↓ Cough	↑ Swelling of feet Tighter-fitting clothes ↑ SOB and DOE ↓ Exercise tolerance More problems sleeping ↑ Cough ↓ Or loss of appetite Nausea Vomiting Halos around lights Yellowish visual tinting Abdominal discomfort Palpitations Weakness Lethargy Agitation or disorientation Muscle cramps Dry mouth Thirst Dizziness Upset stomach Confusion Persistent dry cough Itching Maculopapular or morbilliform rash Dysgeusia Diarrhea

FIGURE 8-11 *Integrated Subjective Parameters Monitoring Plan.* Integrated subjective monitoring plan for digoxin, furosemide, captopril, and potassium chloride.

❚ SELF-ASSESSMENT QUESTIONS ❚

1 Which of the following are needed to monitor patient response to drug therapy?
   a. Knowledge of pharmacotherapeutics
   b. Knowledge of pathophysiology
   c. Communication skills
   d. Physical assessment skills
   e. All of the above

2 Which of the following is the first step in the monitoring process?
   a. Monitor the response to therapy.
   b. Assess the response to therapy.
   c. Set therapeutic goals.
   d. Integrate the monitoring plan.
   e. Determine specific monitoring parameters.

Objective—Therapeutic	Objective—Toxic
↓ Heart size on CXR	↑ Heart size on CXR
↓ Edema on CXR	↑ Edema on CXR
↓ Weight	↑ Weight
↑ Ejection fraction	↓ Ejection fraction
Improved R wave progression	Poor R wave progression
Normalization of S:R	Abnormal S:R on ECG
↓ T wave inversion	↑ T wave inversion
Serum potassium	VPDs
	Arrhythmias on ECG
	Serum digoxin greater than 2 ng/ml
	↓ Heart rate
	↓ Blood pressure
	↓ Serum potassium
	↑ Serum glucose
	↑ Serum uric acid
	↑ Serum BUN/serum creatinine ratio
	↑ Serum BUN
	↑ Serum creatinine
	↑ Heart rate
	U waves or flat or inverted T waves
	↑ Temperature
	Eosinophilia
	Proteinuria
	WBC with differential
	Flattened P waves
	Widened QRS complex
	Peaked T wave

FIGURE 8-12 *Integrated Objective Parameters Monitoring Plan.* Example of integrated objective monitoring plan for digoxin, furosemide, captopril, and potassium chloride.

3 Which of the following is the last step in the monitoring process?
   a. Monitor the response to therapy.
   b. Assess the response to therapy.
   c. Set therapeutic goals.
   d. Integrate the monitoring plan.
   e. Determine specific monitoring parameters.

4 For which kind of patient is the availability of monitoring data limited?
   a. A hospitalized, critically ill patient
   b. A patient just started on insulin therapy
   c. A patient with stable, well-controlled mild hypertension
   d. A patient undergoing renal dialysis
   e. A postsurgical trauma patient

5 For which kind of patient is the largest amount of monitoring data available?
   a. A hospitalized, critically ill patient
   b. A patient just started on insulin therapy
   c. A patient with stable, well-controlled mild hypertension
   d. A patient undergoing renal dialysis
   e. A postsurgical trauma patient

6 A patient is receiving a medication associated with hypokalemia (reference range of 3.5 to 5.5 mEq/L). Which of the following is an appropriate therapeutic goal when monitoring potassium-replacement therapy?
   a. Serum potassium 4.0 mEq/L
   b. Serum potassium greater than 5.5 mEq/L
   c. Serum potassium less than 3.5 mEq/L
   d. Serum potassium 3.5 to 5.5 mEq/L
   e. Serum potassium 2.0 to 3.0 mEq/L

Refer to the following information for questions 7 through 10: A patient with pneumonia is receiving an antibiotic for treatment of acute bronchitis. The patient's symptoms include cough and fever. The antibiotic may cause diarrhea and thrombocytopenia.

7 *Decreased cough* is what type of monitoring parameter?
   a. Subjective-therapeutic
   b. Subjective-toxic
   c. Objective-therapeutic
   d. Objective-toxic
   e. None of the above

8 *Decreased fever* is what type of monitoring parameter?
   a. Subjective-therapeutic
   b. Subjective-toxic
   c. Objective-therapeutic
   d. Objective-toxic
   e. None of the above

9 *Diarrhea* is what type of monitoring parameter?
   a. Subjective-therapeutic
   b. Subjective-toxic
   c. Objective-therapeutic
   d. Objective-toxic
   e. None of the above

10 *Thrombocytopenia* is what type of monitoring parameter?
   a. Subjective-therapeutic
   b. Subjective-toxic
   c. Objective-therapeutic
   d. Objective-toxic
   e. None of the above

CHAPTER 9

Researching and Providing Drug Information

LEARNING OBJECTIVES

1   Identify the components involved in providing drug information to health care professionals and patients.
2   Identify and categorize common types of drug information questions.
3   List examples of questions used to clarify the initial drug information question.
4   State the key to a successful search of the published literature.
5   Differentiate among primary, secondary, and tertiary literature.
6   State the way to evaluate primary, secondary, and tertiary literature.
7   Describe the way to access information in textbooks, files using the AHFS numbering system, *Index Medicus,* computerized databases, and the Internet.
8   List the advantages and disadvantages of using the Internet.
9   Describe the best way to communicate answers to drug information questions.

DISSEMINATION of information regarding medications and other pharmaceuticals is an important responsibility. Patients, physicians, nurses, and other health care professionals depend on pharmacists for accurate and timely information about medications. Drug information commonly includes data regarding drug dosing, availability, and side effects; however, pharmacists often answer a broad range of questions in providing drug information (Box 9-1).

To respond effectively to drug information questions, pharmacists must have good communication skills, knowledge of literature resources and ways to access them, and the ability to evaluate published information. Some questions can be answered by relying on previously acquired knowledge; other questions require a search and assessment of current reference textbooks and medical and pharmacy literature.

THE PROCESS

The important components involved in the provision of drug information include determining the primary question, developing an appropriate search strategy, locating appropriate sources of information if the question cannot be answered from previously acquired knowledge, assessing the available information, and providing a verbal or written response to the question.

Determining the Primary Question

People generally find formulating specific drug information questions difficult. Most questions arise as the result of a patient-specific problem; however, questions often are presented initially as broad-based theoretical problems. For example, a

Box 9-1. *Types of Drug Information Questions*

ADVERSE DRUG REACTIONS
Adverse reactions
Allergies
Teratogenicity
Toxicology

DOSING
Age-specific dosing
Dosing in altered organ function
    (liver, renal)
Indication-specific dosing

DRUG ADMINISTRATION
Commercial dosage form alterations
    (crushing, dissolving)
Drug administration methods
Product preparation (reconstitution,
    admixing, compounding)
Compatibility, stability, and storage
Timing (with or without food or enteral
    products)

DRUG INTERACTIONS
Drug-drug
Drug-food

Drug-laboratory
Drug-nutrient

INDICATIONS AND THERAPEUTIC USE
Approved drugs
Investigational drugs
Unapproved drugs

POISONINGS AND TOXICOLOGY
Signs and symptoms
Treatment

PRODUCT-SPECIFIC CONCERNS
Constituents (sugars, dyes, adjuvants,
    alcohol)
Formulations
Identification
Storage

MISCELLANEOUS
Drug use during pregnancy and lactation
Pharmacoeconomics
Product-specific assays
Veterinary drug information

physician may ask for the incidence of ceftriaxone allergic reactions when in fact the actual question is whether ceftriaxone is the cause of an otherwise unexplained neutropenia in a patient. Patients may have the same difficulty phrasing questions as do health care professionals. For example, many patients do not understand the difference between an allergy and an adverse reaction. Patients may ask about drug allergies when they really want to know whether the medication they are taking is the cause of a specific problem such as nausea, constipation, headache, or drowsiness.

To determine the primary question, the pharmacist needs to ask the person asking the question a number of clarification questions. An important starting point is to ask whether the question pertains to a specific patient and if so to ask for pertinent background patient information. For example, if the question is about the possibility of an adverse reaction in a specific patient, the pharmacist must determine the nature of the suspected problem and obtain details about the patient's current medication regimen, including all drugs, dosages, and duration of therapy. Laboratory and physical examination findings also may be important pertinent details. Questions about therapeutic options may require even more information about the patient's diagnosis and past and current medication regimens.

After the primary question and patient-specific details have been identified, the pharmacist should rephrase and restate the question to confirm that the pharmacist and the person asking the question understand and agree. Clarifying questions should be asked and information exchanged until the primary question is agreed on and enough patient-specific information and other background information are known to allow for a focused search for an answer. The pharmacist may have to review the patient's chart and interview the patient directly to locate all pertinent background patient information.

The pharmacist also has to determine when the answer is needed and the way to contact the person who needs the information. Some questions require immediate responses for urgent patient care decisions; other questions are not as urgent and can be answered later the same day or even several days later. The pharmacist should not assume that every question is urgent and has to be answered immediately at the expense of other responsibilities or that every question can be postponed. The pharmacist should ask for the person's telephone or beeper number or arrange to provide the information face to face at a certain time and place such as in the clinic the next afternoon or during patient rounds later that morning.

Developing an Appropriate Search Strategy

Searching for drug information is a complex process that requires thought before action. A great deal of time can be wasted by searching for information in the wrong places or by searching the on-line literature with inappropriate search terms. Therefore the pharmacist should formulate a strategy for locating the answer to the question.

The key to developing an appropriate search strategy is to think about the question asked and match the question with the most appropriate sources of information. Questions of fact such as dosage formulations, usual dosage regimens, dosage adjustments in renal and hepatic dysfunction, pharmacokinetic parameters for drugs that have been marketed for several years, and spectrum of activities of marketed antibiotics are best answered by looking up the information (either manually or on-line) in standard pharmacy textbooks such as the *American Hospital Formulary Service* (AHFS). Questions about investigational drugs, unapproved indications for currently marketed drugs, and unusual adverse effects and drug interactions are best answered by a thorough literature search (either manually or online) of published medical and pharmacy literature.

The key to a successful search of the published literature is to identify appropriate search terms before starting the search. Terms can sometimes be identified by reading about the topic in a standard medical or pharmacy textbook or published review article; however, the pharmacist may need to look up the terms in the National Library of Medicine's *Medical Subject Headings* (MeSH) book, which identifies key indexing terms for the MEDLINE database. These indexing terms are generally relevant for searches of any medical- or pharmacy-related database.

Flexibility is important when searching for information. If a search does not reveal any relevant information, the cause may be a lack of available information about the subject. More commonly, the literature may not have been searched far enough back in time to locate older information or the search terms were not appropriate. The pharmacist must consider when information about a drug is most likely to have been published and think of additional related indexing terms before deciding that no information about the topic is available in the published literature.

Choosing Sources of Information

Drug information is available verbally from colleagues and other health care professionals and in printed resources such as textbooks and journals. Colleagues may be excellent sources of information; however, their information may be dated or incomplete and is ordinarily without reference. Pharmaceutical companies may be good sources of information about drugs in their product lines. Information may be obtained by written inquiry or more commonly by contacting the company's drug information center or product manager. However, pharmaceutical companies can only provide information regarding labeled indications. Pharmaceutical companies cannot disclose confidential data, nor can they discuss other proprietary information. In addition, the pharmaceutical industry is required by law to compile and report adverse drug reaction information. Therefore if a company receives an inquiry regarding a possible adverse effect associated with one of its products, it is obligated to obtain detailed information about the event and report it to the federal government.

Primary Literature. Primary literature, consisting of original data, research, and case reports, is published in journals, other periodicals, and collections of research presentations and other special proceedings (Box 9-2). The amount of full-text primary literature posted directly on the Internet is growing rapidly. Primary literature generally contains the most recent information available for any given topic.

Although primary literature is published in many different sources, the quality of the information varies greatly. No article can be accepted at face value without a complete assessment of the publication. One initial judge of the quality of a journal is the impact or perceived prestige of the journal. Authors try to have their manuscripts published in journals that have the greatest impact on health care professionals. Therefore a lot of competition for publication in these journals occurs. Articles selected for publication in these journals tend to be well-written manuscripts about high-quality research. Two general indications of quality are the overall reputation of the journal and whether the journal uses a peer-review process.

The impact of journals can be judged by the citation rates for the articles contained within them. In a 1986 report on the impact of medical journals, the *New England Journal of Medicine* and *Lancet* accounted for more than one third of all the 1981 citations.[1] Other frequently cited journals included the *Annals of Internal Medicine*, the *British Medical Journal*, and the *Journal of the American Medical Association*. These are general medical journals; specialty and subspecialty journals have smaller circulations and therefore less impact.

Refereed articles are articles that have undergone peer review before acceptance

---

Box 9-2   *Common Primary Sources of Drug Information*

MEDICAL JOURNALS
General medical journals
American Journal of Medicine
Annals of Internal Medicine
Journal of the American Medical Association
Lancet
New England Journal of Medicine

Specialty medical journals
American Journal of Cardiology
American Journal of Respiratory and Critical Care Medicine
Blood

Circulation
Diabetes
Gastroenterology
Journal of Infectious Disease

PHARMACY AND PHARMACOLOGY JOURNALS
American Journal of Health-System Pharmacy
Annals of Pharmacotherapy
Clinical Pharmacology and Therapeutics
Hospital Pharmacy
Journal of Clinical Pharmacology
Pharmacotherapy

for publication. The editors, after an initial internal review of the manuscript, ask outside experts for a thorough review of the manuscript. Peer review provides expert opinion regarding the originality of the material, validity of the data, appropriateness of the conclusions, and importance and relevance of the information.

Secondary and Tertiary Literature. Secondary and tertiary literature consists of compiled information. This type of literature includes compiled databases, review articles published in journals, symposia published in journal supplements, and textbooks (Box 9-3). Secondary and tertiary literature comprises reviews, analyses, interpretations, assessments, and conclusions made from assessment of multiple

---

Box 9-3 *Common Secondary and Tertiary Sources of Drug Information*

PERIODICALS

Clin-Alert
Facts and Comparisons Drug Newsletter
FDA Medical Bulletin
The Medical Letter
DRUGDEX System
International Pharmaceutical Abstracts
Iowa Drug Information System
POISINDEX System
Unlisted Drugs

TEXTBOOKS

AMA drug evaluations, ed 7, Philadelphia, 1991, WB Saunders.
American drug index, Philadelphia, 1997, Lippincott.
McEvoy GK: *AHFS drug information,* Bethesda, Md, 1997, American Society of Health-System Pharmacists.
Young LY, Koda-Kimble MA: *Applied therapeutics: the clinical use of drugs,* ed 6, Vancouver, Wash, 1996, Applied Therapeutics.
Evans WE, Schentag JJ, Jusko WJ: *Applied pharmacokinetics: principles of therapeutic drug monitoring,* ed 3, Vancouver, Wash, 1992, Applied Therapeutics.
Gosselin RE: *Clinical toxicology of commercial products,* ed 5, Baltimore, 1984, Williams & Wilkins.
Hansten PD, Horn PD: *Hansten and Horn's drug interactions analysis and management,* Vancouver, Wash, 1997, Applied Therapeutics.
Drug facts and comparisons, ed 51, St Louis, 1997, Facts and Comparisons.
Tatro DS: *Drug interactions facts,* ed 5, St Louis, 1996, Facts and Comparisons.
Handbook of antimicrobial therapy, New Rochelle, NY, 1996, Medical Letter.

Anderson PO, Knoben JE: *Handbook of clinical drug data,* ed 8, Stamford, CT, 1997, Appleton & Lange.
Trissel LA: *Handbook on injectable drugs,* ed 9, Bethesda, Md, 1996, American Society of Health System Pharmacists.
Handbook of nonprescription drugs, ed 11, Washington, DC, 1996, American Pharmaceutical Association.
Dreisbach RH, Robertson WO: *Handbook of poisoning: prevention, diagnosis, and treatment,* ed 12, Los Altos, Calif, 1987, Appleton & Lange.
Harrison's principles of internal medicine, ed 14, New York, 1997, McGraw-Hill.
Martindale W: *Martindale: the extra pharmacopoeia,* ed 31, London, 1996, Royal Pharmaceutical Society.
Budavari S: *Merck index,* ed 12, Whitehouse Station, NJ, 1996, Merck.
Dukes MNG: *Meyler's side effects of drugs,* ed 13, Amsterdam, NY, 1996, Elsevier.
DiPiro JT et al: *Pharmacotherapy,* ed 3, Stamford, CT, 1996, Appleton & Lange.
Physician's desk reference, ed 51, Montvale, NJ, 1997, Medical Economics.
Gennaro AR: *Remington's pharmaceutical sciences,* ed 19, Easton, Penn, 1995, Mack.
Unlisted drugs index, ed 9, Chatham, 1992, Unlisted Drugs.
USP drug information, ed 17, Rockville, Md, 1997, United States Pharmacopeia Convention.
Herfindal ET, Gourley DR: *Textbook of therapeutics,* ed 6, Baltimore, 1996, Williams and Wilkins.
The United States pharmacopoeia and the national formulary, ed 23, Rockville, Md, 1995, Board of Trustees (United States Pharmacopeial Convention).

sources of original data. Authors of secondary and tertiary literature may or may not be considered experts in the topic.

The distinction between secondary and tertiary literature is indistinct. Although compiled periodicals and abstracting services are commonly referred to as secondary literature and textbooks and compendia are commonly referred to as tertiary literature, overlap occurs. Secondary literature tends to be slightly more current than tertiary literature but may not be subject to as extensive prepublication review as is tertiary literature.

Textbooks and other published books are the least up-to-date sources of information because publication takes 2 to 3 years and the information contained in a book is out of date by at least that length of time. In addition, the author or authors may have taken a year or more to write the text and a several-year gap may occur between new editions of textbooks, making the information even more out of date.

Secondary and tertiary literature can be a good source of general or overview information about a topic, but it cannot be relied on to provide the most up-to-date information regarding indications, usages, mechanisms of action, adverse effects, and drug interactions for specific drugs. Secondary and tertiary literature may not contain any information about investigational drugs, newly marketed drugs, uncommon side effects and drug interactions, or new indications for previously marketed drugs.

Accessing Printed Sources of Information

Printed sources of information can be accessed by searching the indexes of textbooks, locating articles in individually maintained files of journal article reprints, manually searching for appropriate citations in bibliographic systems such as *Index Medicus,* and using on-line bibliographic and full-text computer services and software. Print resources are located in biomedical libraries. On-line resources are available in most biomedical libraries and may be accessible from any computer with a modem, depending on the service.

Textbooks. Most pharmacists are familiar with locating information using textbook indexes. The key to locating information through textbook indexes is to look for the precise topic and think of synonyms and related terms if the initial topic is not listed.

Individual Files. The location of articles in individually maintained files of journal article reprints depends on the system used to file the articles. Some pharmacists use complex filing strategies. For example, some pharmacists set up their files using the American Hospital Formulary System (AHFS) numbering system. To locate specific topics, the searcher must be familiar with the AHFS or look up the drug topic in the AHFS book. Other pharmacists use simpler but highly individualized topic groupings based on specific disease states, organ systems, or pharmacotherapeutic categories.

Manual Indexes. *Index Medicus* classifies and indexes articles using a set vocabulary of indexing words (MeSH) and a fixed, hierarchic structure (MeSH tree structure). Complete article citations, including author, title, journal, volume, issue, and inclusive page numbers, are published in monthly indexes for the current year and annual indexes for past years. Successful manual searching of *Index Medicus* depends on the selection of appropriate index terms and careful perusal of each volume in the current year and as many annual volumes as necessary to locate the appropriate body of literature about the topic. After appropriate citations have been found, the journal must be located in the holdings of the library. *Index Medicus* indexes more than 3000 journals. Pharmacists may thus retrieve appropriate citations in journals that are not readily available in local pharmacy or medical libraries.

Computerized Databases. The availability of computerized databases has simplified the process of obtaining drug information and greatly expanded access to published information. Examples of health-related databases include MEDLINE (the on-line equivalent of *Index Medicus*), Current Contents, International Pharmaceutical Abstracts (IPA), and Cancerlit. Computerized databases can be searched by librarians as a service for health care professionals or by the person who needs the information (commonly referred to as the *end user*). End-user on-line searching is rapidly becoming the standard of practice as appropriately equipped personal computers are becoming more accessible in patient care areas, drug information centers, medical and pharmacy libraries, offices, and homes.

On-line searching of computerized databases is best suited for specific drug information questions and information about recent topics. Getting a broad-based overview of complex topics is more difficult with on-line searching; textbooks are better sources of information for these types of questions. Many on-line databases were started in the mid-1960s and early 1970s. Therefore information dating earlier than this time usually has to be searched manually.

On-line searching of computerized databases is more efficient than manual searching of indexes because the computer can rapidly search extensive databases. On-line searching of computerized databases is easier than manual searching because the information can be searched using a variety of terms and approaches, including key indexing terms, truncated terms, author, title, and type of publication.

Access to computerized databases is made through public and commercial vendors. The National Library of Medicine (NLM), the creator of MEDLINE, is a public vendor. Dialog Information Services and Bibliographic Retrieval Services (BRS) are commercial vendors.

Two types of information are available to users of computerized databases. First, most databases provide at least the full bibliographic citation, including all authors, title, journal, year, volume number, issue number, and inclusive page numbers. Key indexing terms are listed, which may narrow the search, provide additional search terms, and suggest related topics. Second, the manuscript abstract may be provided if available. Some of the databases provide the full text of the manuscripts contained in the database; other databases provide the full text of a variety of pharmacy and medical textbooks. Generally, the information can be downloaded and printed on the user's printer.

On-line searching requires access to a computer, modem, communications software, and a knowledge of ways to access computerized databases. Some training is required to learn to use the search programs; however, user-friendly programs requiring minimal training are available.

On-line searching may be quite expensive, depending on the annual fee for access to the service and the charge for each search. The fee for each search depends on the amount of time connected to the database, amount of processing the computer must do to accomplish the search, number of characters printed, and time of day.

The Internet. Searchable databases are limited to previously published information. This limit confers a certain degree of reliability but restricts access to specific types of information. Although the availability of full-text publications is increasing, information in the databases is usually limited to published abstracts. In addition, some delay (weeks to months) always occurs between publication in the print media and inclusion of the information in the database. In contrast, information on the Internet is completely unrestricted and access is nearly instantaneous.

The Internet, consisting of thousands of connected computer networks, provides access to a wide array of information, including information traditionally published in newsletters, magazines, journals, newspapers, and books, and access to live discussion groups, sound, and video images. Government health agencies, international health organizations, pharmaceutical companies, and professional organizations also post information on the Internet.[2,3] One clear advantage of the Internet is the connection of information through cross-listings and links that provide rapid access to related information on the Internet.

Access to information on the Internet requires a computer, modem, telephone line, access to a provider service, and specific networking and application software computer programs. The primary advantage of the Internet (access to a vast array of unlimited and uncontrolled information) also is its greatest disadvantage; no limits are placed on information posted on the Internet. No person or group controls the Internet, no universal indexing system is available, and no quality controls are placed on information. Therefore finding information may be time consuming and frustrating. In addition, after the information has been located, no assurances are made as to its validity and reliability.

Information can be retrieved using search engines, software programs that index and search Internet resources. Yahoo!, Lycos, Infoseek, WAIS (wide area information servers), and HotBot are search engines. Search engines locate information by searching for specific terms and phrases; links between terms can be made using Boolean logic (such as and, or, not). Search results are displayed in ranked lists according to the degree to which the terms and topics match; specific information is located by opening and reading the content of the lists. Because search engines differ in the scope of Internet sources searched, the pharmacist may wish to search the Internet using more than one search engine.

Locating inaccurate or false information on the Internet is a risk. The risk can be lowered by limiting searches to generally reputable sources such as government agencies and using sources that provide references for the information.

Critical Appraisal of Information Sources

After information has been located, it cannot be used at face value without critical appraisal of its source. All information, including textbooks, review articles published in refereed and nonrefereed journals, and original research articles, must be evaluated critically for timeliness, reliability, and applicability before the information is used to answer a question.

Textbooks. Information obtained from textbooks should be evaluated from several different perspectives. The publication date should be noted. Older texts (texts published more than 4 or 5 years ago) may contain information that was correct at time of publication but is inaccurate based on currently available information. This is especially true for pharmacotherapeutics, pathophysiology, pharmacology, and other medically related textbooks. Textbooks also may contain errors. No information should be taken at face value without verification.

The pharmacist should note the author of the chapter or book and judge whether the author has the expertise and experience necessary to be an authoritative source of information. Authors should be practitioners who deal regularly with the issues they are writing about and are familiar with the literature and state-of-the-art issues relevant to the topic. All information obtained from textbooks should be cross-checked if possible with information from a second, more recent source of information.

Literature Reviews. Literature reviews, also known as *review articles,* are published in refereed and nonrefereed journals, special supplements to journals, and other published formats. Literature reviews are information sources somewhat intermediary between original research and textbooks. However, literature reviews must be carefully evaluated[4-6] (Box 9-4). As with textbooks, the pharmacist must judge the currency of the articles by checking the date of publication. Judging the expertise of the author or authors is another important step in reviewing an article.

The pharmacist must assess the way the authors selected and evaluated the primary research used as the basis of the review. The purpose of the review should be clearly spelled out in the introduction. Because the conclusions of the review article are based on information obtained from relevant original research, the methodology used to locate the research publications should be identified and outlined. Data obtained from previous review articles should not be used; the authors should locate and assess relevant original data, not another person's interpretation of the data. The criteria for extraction and acceptance of data from the original research should be specific and well documented. An assessment should be made regarding whether the conclusions made by the authors of the review reflect the supporting data.

Original Research. Published original research, primarily in the form of clinical trials, is an important source of drug information. Research reports are often quoted as proving the usefulness of specific therapeutic agents for new or unapproved indications and as the basis for proving or disproving the association between a drug and a specific adverse drug reaction or interaction. However, original research articles must be carefully evaluated (Box 9-5). The results as stated by the authors cannot be accepted at face value; a thorough and critical appraisal of the research methodology must be completed before the information can be accepted and used for patient care decisions. A single study cannot stand alone in changing clinical practice. Ideally, multiple studies of different patient populations are needed to change clinical practice.[7]

The validity and applicability of the research must be carefully assessed.[7-9] Validity refers to the likelihood that the study results are true. Applicability refers to the likelihood that the study results can be useful for clinical decision making. The

---

Box 9-4	*Questions to Ask when Reviewing Review Articles*

1. What are the qualifications of the authors?
2. Was the question clearly stated?
3. Were relevant studies located using a comprehensive search strategy?
4. Were the selection criteria used to select studies explicit and clearly identified?

5. Was each study valid?
6. Were study results combined appropriately?
7. Were the conclusions supported by the combined data?

Box 9-5 *Questions to Ask when Reviewing Original Research*

1. What are the qualifications of the investigators?
2. Who funded the study?
3. What are the study's objectives?
4. What is the study design? Is the study design appropriate for the stated objectives?
5. Is a control group being used, and if so, is the control group appropriate for the stated objectives?
6. What are the outcome measures? Are the outcome measures appropriate for the stated objectives?
7. Are the data complete? Are all study subjects accounted for? Are any of the data missing?
8. Were the analytical (laboratory) techniques appropriate for the type of samples?
9. Were the statistical analyses appropriate?
10. Are statistically significant results clinically important?
11. Could any uncontrolled factors (such as seasonal variations in severity of disease) have influenced the outcome of the study?
12. What is the clinical relevance of the study results?

---

pharmacist must consider characteristics (e.g., age, sex, severity and duration of disease) of the subjects or patients evaluated in the study and decide if they are similar to those of the patient in question. Although most studies have flaws, useful information can still be obtained by considering the pros and cons and limits of the study.

Critical appraisal of original research begins with a review of the abstract. Abstracts usually contain enough information to determine whether the study applies to the question at hand and is valid enough to merit further evaluation. Structured abstracts in which the objective, study design, setting, subjects, interventions, main outcome measures, results, and conclusions are clearly identified and summarized allow the reader to determine quickly the potential applicability and usefulness of the study.[10]

The objectives of the study should be identified. The objective, a statement of the facts the authors tried to determine, should be stated in the introductory portion of the paper. One of the key components of critical appraisal of original research is to determine whether the authors conducted a study appropriately designed to accomplish the objectives.

The basic study design should be noted and evaluated for appropriateness in the context of the objectives of the study. For example, interventional studies, commonly used to compare drug regimens, are typically randomized or nonrandomized control trials. These types of studies can be blinded or nonblinded, placebo or active controlled, and crossover or parallel in design. The pharmacist must note whether patient adherence to study requirements (such as medication, diet, exercise) was assessed and the way adherence was assessed.

The setting of the study should be noted and evaluated for appropriateness in context of the objectives of the study. For example, although flaws are associated with multicenter trials, they are the most appropriate study design for evaluation of treatment options for rare or unusual disease states.

The characteristics of the study participants should be noted and evaluated for appropriateness in context of the objectives of the study. The pharmacist should note the way the study participants were selected and whether the study population is a representative sample. Consideration of whether the study used normal volunteers or patients and was conducted in an inpatient or outpatient setting is an important step in the review process. The pharmacist should consider the median age and range of ages included in the study, the gender distribution of the subjects, and the socioeconomic features of the study population. Explanations of the number of subjects who withdrew and their reasons should be noted; all subjects enrolled in a study should be accounted for in the results.

Assessment of the outcome measures for the study is the next step. The pharmacist should note whether the outcome measures were appropriate for the objectives of the study and whether the parameters used to measure the outcomes were appropriate, comprehensive, and clinically applicable to the study objectives.

The study results should be reviewed in detail. The pharmacist should review the data contained in the tables, graphs, and charts in detail to verify the authors conclusions and note whether the published conclusions are supported by the data and the statistical analyses are appropriate for the study design and types of data. Finally, the pharmacist should determine whether the study results, even if they are statistically significant, are clinically significant.

Answering the Question

After the information has been located and analyzed, the answer to the question can be formulated and conveyed to the person asking the question. An answer may be as simple as a specific dosage or may require an extensive search for information and the assessment and synthesis of numerous original research articles. In either case the answer must be timely, concise, precise, appropriate to the background of the person asking the question, and referenced.

The quality and accuracy of the answer depend on the quality and validity of the search strategy and documents used to formulate the answer. Verification of the answer in more than one documented source of information adds confidence that the information provided is accurate.

Verbal communication of drug information must be clear and fluent. The information should be well organized with an appropriate emphasis on important details. The information should be conveyed with confidence and at a level appropriate to the questioner. The pharmacist should be able to expand on the information according to the needs of the questioner.

Written communication of drug information must be well organized, complete, and well written. Appropriate sentence and paragraph structure and correct grammar, punctuation, and spelling should be used. References should be complete and in a uniformly accepted format such as that described in the "Uniform Requirements for Manuscripts Submitted to Biomedical Journals."[11]

The written response includes a statement of the question, relevant patient details (such as age, disease history, drug history), relevant data from the literature sources, evaluation of the literature cited, summary, conclusions and recommendations, and references. The written response should flow well with smooth transitions between sections. The name of the person asking the question and the name of the person answering the question should be documented on the written response.

The question, answer, and references used to determine the answer should be documented for future reference. In some situations (such as in drug information centers) a written response to a question must be documented. In some cases the question and response are documented in the patient's clinic record or chart.

DRUG INFORMATION CENTERS

More than 200 pharmacist-operated drug information centers are in operation in the United States.[12] Most of these centers are located in hospitals and run by the hospital's pharmacy department. However, some drug information centers are located in medical libraries, colleges of pharmacy, and poison control centers. Most pharmaceutical companies have in-house drug information centers.[13]

The University of Kentucky Drug Information Center was the first drug information center in the United States. It began operation in 1962 as a drug information source, an aid to teaching, an aid in the selection and rational use of drugs, a center for reporting adverse drug reactions, a stimulus for the development of additional drug information centers, and a training site for drug information specialists.[14] These tasks remain the focus of most drug information centers today. The primary activities of drug information centers include drug information activities; formulary activities; publication of newsletters and other related publications; staff development; investigational drug program activities; drug use review, adverse drug reaction reporting; research; and training of students, pharmacy residents, and drug information specialists.

A variety of drug information questions are routinely handled by drug information centers. Questions include indications, dosages, side effects, metabolism, availability, toxicity, interactions, contraindications, pharmaceutical compatibility, pharmacokinetic calculations, and identification of American and international products.

Drug information specialists are pharmacists who have received specialized training in drug information, generally in the form of 1-year residency programs in drug information provided by hospitals and other drug information centers. Drug information specialists are skilled in locating and evaluating drug information and communicating with pharmacists, physicians, other health care providers, and patients.

SELF-ASSESSMENT QUESTIONS

1 Which of the following are important components involved in the provision of drug information?
   a. Determining the primary question
   b. Developing an appropriate search strategy
   c. Assessing available information
   d. All of the above
   e. None of the above

2 A consumer asks whether her new prescription drug is the cause of her insomnia. What type of drug information question is this?
   a. Adverse reaction
   b. Dosing

    c. Drug administration
    d. Indication and therapeutic use
    e. Poisoning and toxicology

3 A colleague asks if ipratropium bromide (Atrovent) is FDA approved for the treatment of asthma. What type of drug information question is this?
    a. Adverse reaction
    b. Dosing
    c. Drug administration
    d. Indication and therapeutic use
    e. Poisoning and toxicology

4 Which one of the following is an example of primary literature?
    a. An original study published in the *New England Journal of Medicine*
    b. A review of a newly marketed drug published in the *Medical Letter*
    c. A drug interaction described in a drug interactions book

5 Which one of the following is an example of secondary literature?
    a. An original study published in the *New England Journal of Medicine*
    b. A review of a newly marketed drug published in the *Medical Letter*
    c. A drug interaction described in a drug interactions book

6 Which one of the following is an example of tertiary literature?
    a. An original study published in the *New England Journal of Medicine*
    b. A review of a newly marketed drug published in the *Medical Letter*
    c. A drug interaction described in a drug interactions book

7 Which of the following are important considerations when evaluating an original research article?
    a. Appropriateness of the study design
    b. Clinical significance of statistically significant data
    c. Study participant characteristics
    d. All of the above
    e. None of the above

8 Which of the following are important considerations when evaluating a literature review?
    a. Publication date
    b. Author expertise
    c. Way the author selected the primary research articles
    d. All of the above
    e. None of the above

9 Which of the following is the most appropriate source of information regarding questions of fact such as usual dosage regimens?
    a. The pharmaceutical company
    b. A colleague
    c. A standard pharmacy textbook
    d. An on-line search of the published literature
    e. All of the above

10 Which of the following is the most appropriate source of information regarding an unapproved indication for a currently marketed drug?
    a. The pharmaceutical company

b. A colleague
c. A standard pharmacy textbook
d. An on-line search of the published literature
e. All of the above

REFERENCES

1. Garfield E: Which medical journals have the greatest impact? *Ann Intern Med* 105:313-320, 1986.
2. Marra CA et al: Drug and poison information resources on the Internet, Part 1: an introduction, *Pharmacotherapy* 16:537-546, 1996.
3. Marra CA et al: Drug and poison information resources on the Internet, Part 2: identification and evaluation, *Pharmacotherapy* 16:806-818, 1996.
4. Morgan PP: Review articles: 1. Looking over the field, *Can Med Assoc J* 134:11, 1986.
5. Morgan PP: Review articles: 2. The literature jungle, *Can Med Assoc J* 134:98-99, 1986.
6. Oxman AD, Guyatt GH: Guidelines for reading literature reviews, *Can Med Assoc J* 138:697-703, 1988.
7. Weintraub M: How to evaluate reports of clinical trials, *P & T* 17:1463-1473, 1990.
8. Fowkes FGR, Fulton PM: Critical appraisal of published research: introductory guidelines, *Br Med J* 302:1136-1140, 1991.
9. Gardner MJ, Machin D, Campbell MJ: Use of check lists in assessing the statistical content of medical studies, *Br Med J* 292:810-812, 1986.
10. Haynes RB et al: More informative abstracts revisited, *Ann Intern Med* 113:69-76, 1990.
11. International Committee of Medical Journal Editors: Uniform requirements for manuscripts submitted to biomedical journals, *N Engl J Med* 324:424-428, 1991.
12. Beaird SL, Coley RMR, Crea KA: Current status of drug information centers, *Am J Hosp Pharm* 49:103-106, 1992.
13. Colvin CL: Understanding the resources and organization of an industry-based drug information service, *Am J Hosp Pharm* 47:1989-1990, 1990.
14. Parker PF: The University of Kentucky Drug Information Center, *Am J Hosp Pharm* 22:42-47, 1965.

CHAPTER 10

Ethics in Pharmacy and Health Care

LEARNING OBJECTIVES

1 Identify the fundamental moral principle on which all ethical behavior is based.
2 Describe the commonalities among the pharmacy, medical, and nursing codes of ethics.
3 Describe the intent and content of the Patient's Bill of Rights.
4 List actions pharmacists should take to uphold patient confidentiality.
5 Identify the two internationally recognized research codes of ethics.
6 State the composition and responsibilities of research review boards.
7 Identify the required and optional elements of informed consent.
8 Describe two ethical implications of accepting gifts from the pharmaceutical industry.
9 Differentiate between the purposes of living wills and durable powers of attorney.
10 State at least one advantage and disadvantage of living wills and durable powers of attorney.

ETHICS is the science of morality. All ethical behavior is based on the fundamental moral principle of doing good and avoiding evil. Ethical behavior in the profession of pharmacy also means conforming with the rules governing the rights and duties of pharmacists, patients, and other health professionals.

Health professionals grapple with numerous ethical issues (Box 10-1). Some issues such as assisted suicide and assisted reproduction are of interest to health professionals in general but have minimal impact on the daily practice of pharmacy. Other issues such as confidentiality and withholding or withdrawing specific therapeutic interventions commonly influence the practice of pharmacy.

This chapter identifies and describes the professional codes of ethics that form the basis of professional ethical behavior and discusses several specific ethical issues, including confidentiality, research ethics, ethics and the promotion of drugs, and the use of advance directives in end-of-life decisions. Additional information regarding biomedical ethical principles is available in biomedical ethics textbooks. Detailed specific discussions regarding biomedical ethical issues are published in the medical literature; discussions of specific dispensing-related ethical issues are published in the pharmacy literature.

PROFESSIONAL CODES OF ETHICS

Most health professions have specific codes of ethics that provide written guidelines regarding ethical behavior. The medical code of ethics, often considered the foundation for ethical behavior in health care, dates to the time of Hippocrates; other codes of ethics are more recent. Most professional codes of ethics are written

Box 10-1 *Examples of Health Care–Related Ethical Issues*

Abortifacients (RU486, antiprogestins)	Risk/benefit limitations (e.g., in clozapine
Assisted reproduction and donation of	therapy)
genetic material	Substance abuse and dependence
Confidentiality	Withholding or withdrawing treatment in-
Euthanasia and assisted suicide	terventions
Performance enhancers	Cardiopulmonary resuscitation
Research	Fluids
Animal testing	Intubation and ventilation
Biologic research	Nutrition (tube feedings, total parenteral
Genetic research	nutrition)
Informed consent	
Investigational drugs	

using broad-based directives that do not provide issue-specific guidelines. This means that the ethical guidelines for most health professionals are deliberately vague. Therefore to be ethical requires that health professionals apply their professional codes of ethics within a framework of societal moral values. Individual philosophies and beliefs must be considered and respected.

The Hippocratic Oath

The Hippocratic oath, attributed to the fifth century BC Greek physician Hippocrates, is considered the basis for modern medical ethical standards.[1] The oath is found in the Hippocratic corpus, a collection of literature containing case reports, descriptions of disease processes, and medical philosophies generally attributed to Hippocrates. Issues addressed in the oath include patient advocacy, patient confidentiality, professional misconduct, and the need to defer to those with more appropriate training and experience (Box 10-2).

The Pharmacy Code of Ethics

The foundation of ethical pharmacy behavior is the premise that the welfare of humanity is the pharmacist's primary consideration. The declaration that "Every pharmacist shall devote himself carefully and diligently to his task so that the sick and suffering are not neglected and no harm is done to them" was made by a group of pharmacists in 1456.[2] The document containing this statement is considered one of the oldest known ethical commitments made by a group of pharmacists.

The first American pharmacy code of ethics was adopted in 1848 by the Philadelphia College of Pharmacy.[3] This early pharmacy code of ethics states the responsibility of the pharmacist to the patient and recognizes the professional relationship between pharmacists and physicians. The preface to the code includes the following statement:[3]

> Pharmacy being a profession which demands knowledge, skill, and integrity on the part of those engaged in it, and being associated with the medical profession in the responsible duties of preserving the public health, and dispensing the useful though often dangerous agents adapted to the cure of disease, its members should be united on some general principle to be observed in their several relations to each other, to the medical profession, and to the public.

Box 10-2	*The Hippocratic Oath*

I swear by Apollo Physician and Aesculapius and Hygeia and Panacea and all the gods and goddesses, making them my witnesses, that I will fulfill according to my ability and judgment this oath and this covenant:

To hold him who has taught me this art as equal to my parents and to live my life in partnership with him, and if he is in need of money to give him a share of mine, and to regard his offspring as equal to my brothers in male lineage and to teach them this art— if they desire to learn it—without fee and covenant; to give a share of precepts and oral instruction and all the other learning to my sons and to the sons of him who has instructed me and to pupils who have signed the covenant and have taken an oath according to medical law, but to no one else.

I will apply dietetic measures for the benefit of the sick according to my ability and judgment; I will keep them from harm and injustice.

I will neither give a deadly drug to anybody if asked for it, nor will I make a suggestion to this effect. Similarly I will not give to a woman an abortive remedy. In purity and holiness I will guard my life and my art.

I will not use the knife, not even on sufferers from stone, but will withdraw in favor of such men as are engaged in this work.

Whatever houses I may visit, I will come for the benefit of the sick, remaining free from all intentional injustice, of all mischief and in particular of sexual relations with both female and male persons, be they free or slaves.

What I may see or hear in the course of the treatment or even outside of the treatment in regard to the life of men, which on no account one must spread abroad, I will keep to myself holding such things shameful to be spoken about.

If I fulfill this oath and do not violate it, may it be granted to me to enjoy life and art, be honored with fame among all men for all time to come; if I transgress it and swear falsely, may the opposite of all this be my lot.

Modified from Temkin O, Temkin CL: *Ancient medicine: selected papers of Ludwig Edelstein,* Baltimore, 1967, Johns Hopkins University.

Additional components of the code address the need for reasonable remuneration for services and products, the need to distinguish between pure and impure drugs, the need to control the distribution of poisons, and the minimum requirements for education and apprenticeship.

The American Pharmaceutical Association (APhA), founded in 1852, modeled its first code of ethics after the Philadelphia College of Pharmacy code of ethics. Generally accepted as the professional guidelines for American pharmacists, the APhA code of ethics was revised in 1922, 1952, 1969, 1975, and 1994. The 1994 code of ethics (Box 10-3) differs significantly from earlier codes in that it provides principles based on "moral obligations and virtues" rather than practice-specific guidelines.[4] The 1994 code for the first time defined the pharmacist-patient relationship as a covenant, implying moral obligations such as compassion, caring, honesty, and integrity.[5]

The duty to accept the profession's ethical principles is further emphasized by the oath of the pharmacist[6] (Box 10-4). The oath, traditionally taken at the time of graduation from pharmacy school, states that the primary concern of the pharmacist is the welfare of humanity and relief of human suffering and the pharmacist is expected to maintain the highest standards of moral and ethical conduct.

| Box 10-3 | *The Code of Ethics for Pharmacists* |

PREAMBLE

Pharmacists are health professionals who assist individuals in making the best use of medications. This Code, prepared and supported by pharmacists, is intended to state publicly the principles that form the fundamental basis of the roles and responsibilities of pharmacists. These principles, based on moral obligations and virtues, are established to guide pharmacists in relationships with patients, health professionals, and society.

PRINCIPLES

I. A pharmacist respects the covenantal relationship between the patient and pharmacist.

II. A pharmacist promotes the good of every patient in a caring, compassionate, and confidential manner.

III. A pharmacist respects the autonomy and dignity of each patient.

IV. A pharmacist acts with honesty and integrity in professional relationships.

V. A pharmacist maintains professional competence.

VI. A pharmacist respects the values and abilities of colleagues and other health professionals.

VII. A pharmacist serves individual, community, and societal needs.

VIII. A pharmacist seeks justice in the distribution of health resources.

From *Code of ethics for pharmacists,* Washington, DC, 1995, American Pharmaceutical Association.

| Box 10-4 | *Oath of a Pharmacist* |

At this time, I vow to devote my professional life to the service of all humankind through the profession of pharmacy.

I will consider the welfare of humanity and relief of human suffering my primary concerns.

I will apply my knowledge, experience, and skills to the best of my ability to assure optimal drug therapy outcomes for the patients I serve.

I will keep abreast of developments and maintain professional competency in my profession of pharmacy.

I will maintain the highest principles of moral, ethical, and legal conduct.

I will embrace and advocate change in the profession of pharmacy that improves patient care.

I take these vows voluntarily with the full realization of the responsibility with which I am entrusted by the public.

From *Oath of a pharmacist,* Alexandria, VA, 1995, American Association of Colleges of Pharmacy.

Physician and Nursing Codes of Ethics

The American Medical Association established the first American medical code of ethics in 1847. The code was first revised in 1906 after several decades of discussion and turmoil.[7] The current code, revised in 1992, notes the responsibilities of the physician to patients, society, other health professionals, and self and establishes specific standards of conduct[8] (Box 10-5).

The Florence Nightingale Pledge was written in 1893 by a group of nurses in Detroit (Box 10-6).[9] The American Nurses Association adopted its first code in

| **Box 10-5** | *American Medical Association Principles of Medical Ethics* |

PREAMBLE:

The medical profession has long subscribed to a body of ethical statements developed primarily for the benefit of the patient. As a member of this profession, a physician must recognize responsibility not only to patients, but also to society, to other health professionals, and to self. The following Principles adopted by the American Medical Association are not laws, but standards of conduct which define the essentials of honorable behavior for the physician.

I. A physician shall be dedicated to providing competent medical service with compassion and respect for human dignity.

II. A physician shall deal honestly with patients and colleagues, and strive to expose those physicians deficient in character or competence, or who engage in fraud or deception.

III. A physician shall respect the law and also recognize a responsibility to seek changes in those requirements which are contrary to the best interests of the patient.

IV. A physician shall respect the rights of patients, of colleagues, and of other health professionals, and shall safeguard patient confidences within the constraints of the law.

V. A physician shall continue to study, apply and advance scientific knowledge, make relevant information available to patients, colleagues, and the public, obtain consultation, and use the talents of other health professionals when indicated.

VI. A physician shall, in the provision of appropriate patient care, except in emergencies, be free to chose whom to serve, with whom to associate, and the environment in which to provide medical services.

VII. A physician shall recognize a responsibility to participate in activities contributing to an improved community.

From American Medical Association Council of Ethical and Judicial Affairs: *Current opinion of the Council on Ethical and Judicial Affairs of the American Medical Association,* Chicago, 1992, American Medical Association.

| **Box 10-6** | *The Florence Nightingale Pledge* |

I solemnly pledge myself before God and in the presence of this assembly:

To pass my life in purity and to practice my profession faithfully;

I will abstain from whatever is deleterious and mischievous and will not take or knowingly administer any harmful drug;

I will do all in my power to maintain and elevate the standard of my profession and will hold in confidence all personal matters committed to my keeping and all family affairs coming to my knowledge in the practice of my calling;

With loyalty will I endeavor to aid the physician in his work, and devote myself to the welfare of those committed to my care.

From Kelly C: *Dimensions of professional nursing,* New York, 1962, Macmillan.

1950[10]; the International Code of Nursing Ethics was adopted in 1953.[9] All three documents address confidentiality and commitment to the welfare of patients.

The Patient's Bill of Rights

The patient's bill of rights, affirmed by the American Hospital Association board of trustees in 1972 and revised in 1992, was created to advise hospitalized patients of their rights (Box 10-7).[11] Patients are autonomous and have the right both ethi-

| **Box 10-7** | *A Patient's Bill of Rights** |

1. The patient has the right to considerate and respectful care.
2. The patient has the right to and is encouraged to obtain from physicians and other direct care-givers relevant, current, and understandable information concerning diagnosis, treatment, and prognosis.

    Except in emergencies when the patient lacks decision-making capacity and the need for treatment is urgent, the patient is entitled to the opportunity to discuss and request information related to the specific procedures and/or treatments, the risks involved, the possible length of recuperation, and the medically reasonable alternatives and their accompanying risks and benefits.

    Patients have the right to know the identity of physicians, nurses, and others involved in their care, as well as when those involved are students, residents, or other trainees. The patient also has the right to know the immediate and long-term financial implications of treatment choices, insofar as they are known.
3. The patient has the right to make decisions about the plan of care prior to and during the course of treatment and to refuse a recommended treatment plan of care to the extent permitted by law and hospital policy and to be informed of the medical consequences of this action. In case of such refusal, the patient is entitled to other appropriate care and services that the hospital provides or transfer to another hospital. The hospital should notify patients of any policy that might affect patient choices within the institution.
4. The patient has the right to have an advance directive (such as a living will, health care proxy, or durable power of attorney for health care) concerning treatment or designating a surrogate decision maker with the expectation that the hospital will honor the intent of that directive to the extent permitted by law and hospital policy.

    Health care institutions must advise patients of their rights under state law and hospital policy to make informed medical choices, ask if the patient has an advance directive, and include that information in patient records. The patient has the right to timely information about hospital policy that may limit its ability to implement fully a legally valid advance directive.
5. The patient has the right to every consideration of privacy. Case discussion, consultation, examination, and treatment should be conducted so as to protect each patient's privacy.
6. The patient has the right to expect that all communications and records pertaining to his/her care will be treated as confidential by the hospital, except in cases such as suspected abuse and public health hazards when reporting is permitted or required by law. The patient has the right to expect that the hospital will emphasize the confidentiality of this information when it releases it to any other parties entitled to review information in these records.
7. The patient has the right to review the records pertaining to his/her medical care and to have the information explained or interpreted as necessary, except when restricted by law.
8. The patient has the right to expect that, within its capacity and policies, a hospital will make reasonable response to the request of a patient for appropriate and medically indicated care and services. The hospital must provide evaluation, service, and/or referral as indicated by the urgency of the case. When medically appropriate and legally permissible, or when a patient has so requested, a patient

---

*These rights can be exercised on the patient's behalf by a designated surrogate or proxy decision maker if the patient lacks decision-making capacity, is legally incompetent, or is a minor.

Box 10-7   *A Patient's Bill of Rights—cont'd*

may be transferred to another facility. The institution to which the patient is to be transferred must first have accepted the patient for transfer. The patient must also have the benefit of complete information and explanation concerning the need for, risks, benefits, and alternatives to such a transfer.

9. The patient has the right to ask and be informed of the existence of business relationships among the hospital, educational institutions, other health care providers, or payers that may influence the patient's treatment and care.

10. The patient has the right to consent to or decline to participate in proposed research studies or human experimentation affecting care and treatment or requiring direct patient involvement, and to have those studies fully explained prior to consent. A patient who declines to participate in research or experimentation is entitled to the most effective care that the hospital can otherwise provide.

11. The patient has the right to expect reasonable continuity of care when appropriate and to be informed by physicians and other caregivers of available and realistic patient care options when hospital care is no longer appropriate.

12. The patient has the right to be informed of hospital policies and practices that relate to patient care, treatment, and responsibilities. The patient has the right to be informed of available resources for resolving disputes, grievances and conflicts, such as ethics committees, patient representatives, or other mechanisms available in the institution. The patient has the right to be informed of the hospital's charges for services and available payment methods.

The collaborative nature of health care requires that patients, or their families/ surrogates, participate in their care. The effectiveness of care and patient satisfaction with the course of treatment depend, in part, on the patient fulfilling certain responsibilities. Patients are responsible for providing information about past illnesses, hospitalizations, medications, and other matters related to health status. To participate effectively in decision making, patients must be encouraged to take responsibility for requesting additional information or clarification about their health status or treatment when they do not fully understand information and instructions. Patients are also responsible for ensuring that the health care institution has a copy of their written advance directive if they have one. Patients are responsible for informing their physicians and other caregivers if they anticipate problems in following prescribed treatment.

Patients should also be aware of the hospital's obligation to be reasonably efficient and equitable in providing care to other patients and the community. The hospital's rules and regulations are designed to help the hospital meet this obligation. Patients and their families are responsible for making reasonable accommodations to the needs of the hospital, other patients, medical staff, and hospital employees. Patients are responsible for providing necessary information for insurance claims and for working with the hospital to make payment arrangements, when necessary.

A person's health depends on much more than health care services. Patients are responsible for recognizing the impact of their life-style on their personal health.

CONCLUSION

Hospitals have many functions to perform, including the enhancement of health status, health promotion, and the prevention and treatment of injury and disease; the immediate and ongoing care and rehabilitation of patients; the education of health professionals, patients, and the community; and research. All these activities must be conducted with an overriding concern for the values and dignity of patients.

From *The patient's bill of rights*, Chicago, 1992, American Hospital Association.

cally and legally to make decisions regarding their health care. However, patients may lose the sense of autonomy when hospitalized and may not understand their rights as individuals. The patient's bill of rights recognizes that the institution has a legal responsibility to the patient and a unique relationship with individual patients; it also recognizes the responsibilities of patients. The basic premise of the patient's bill of rights is that all activities must be conducted with an overriding concern for the patient and recognition of the patient's dignity as a human being.

ETHICAL ISSUES

Guidelines for some ethical issues are well established and apply equally to all health professionals. Examples include the ethics of patient confidentiality and clinical research. Some ethical issues such as the relationship between the pharmaceutical industry and health care professionals are relatively new; ethical guidelines are in the process of being formulated and approved. Other issues such as the role of the pharmacist in decisions regarding discontinuation of medical treatment are just being identified; ethical guidelines may take years to develop.

Confidentiality

Confidentiality of patient information is a common ethical issue that all health professionals address daily. The moral concept of confidentiality is present in many religious philosophies and was initially documented for the medical profession in the Hippocratic oath. The Hippocratic oath states that "What I may see or hear in the course of treatment or even outside of the treatment in regard to the life of men, which on no account one must spread abroad, I will keep to myself holding such things shameful to be spoken about."[1] Most health professions provide guidelines regarding confidentiality of patient information.

Confidentiality of patient information must be maintained not only out of respect for the basic moral right of the patient to privacy but also to encourage patients to entrust pharmacists with the details of their illnesses and uses of medications. An environment must be created ensuring patients that information discussed with the pharmacist will be used only by those involved in their care. Few patients would be willing to admit to noncompliance with prescribed medication regimens or would discuss drug abuse if they thought the information would become public.

To uphold patient confidentiality, pharmacists must restrict access to written and computerized patient records, including medication histories and monitoring records. Pharmacists must not discuss specific patient cases in public areas. Discussions with patients and discussions about specific patient cases should be held in private settings. Community pharmacists should use private consultation rooms. Institution-based pharmacists should use conference rooms and other private areas. All pharmacists should avoid discussing patient case information in public areas such as hallways, elevators, and cafeterias.

Research Ethics

Research is an important activity for many pharmacists. Pharmacists frequently serve as principal investigators or coinvestigators. Other research-related responsibilities include protocol development and locating sources of funding, administrative responsibilities such as obtaining institutional approval for research, enrolling subjects, obtaining informed consent, dispensing, inventory control, obtaining data, data analysis, and reporting results.

The need for universally accepted applicable ethical standards evolved as types of research expanded and numbers of research protocols and subjects increased. Historical misconduct added to the need for universal ethical standards. For example, research in the mid-twentieth century often was conducted on prisoners, mentally incompetent persons, and patients in insane asylums; little consideration was given to the ethics of such research or the rights of the participants, who were often viewed as less than human.[12] Nazi abuses of prisoners during World War II led to the development of the Nuremberg code, an internationally recognized research code of ethics (Box 10-8).[13] The World Medical Association Declaration of Helsinki, derived from the Nuremberg Code, is a widely accepted international code of research ethics (Box 10-9).[14]

Box 10-8 *The Nuremberg Code*

The great weight of evidence before us is to the effect that certain types of medical experiments on human beings, when kept within reasonably well-defined bounds, conform to the ethics of the medical profession generally. The protagonists of the practice of human experimentation justify their views on the basis that such experiments yield results for the good of society that are unprocurable by other methods or means of study. All agree, however that certain basic principles must be observed in order to satisfy moral, ethical and legal concepts.

1. The voluntary consent of the human subject is absolutely essential.
2. The experiment should be such as to yield fruitful results for the good of society, unprocurable by other methods or means of study, and not random and unnecessary in nature.
3. The experiment should be so designed and based on the results of animal experimentation and a knowledge of the natural history of the disease or other problem under study that the anticipated results will justify the performance of the experiment.
4. The experiment should be so conducted as to avoid all unnecessary physical and mental suffering and injury.
5. No experiment should be conducted where there is an *a priori* reason to believe that death or disabling injury will occur; except, perhaps, in those experiments where the experimental physicians also serve as subjects.
6. The degree of risk to be taken should never exceed that determined by the humanitarian importance of the problem to be solved by the experiment.
7. Proper preparations should be made and adequate facilities provided to protect the experimental subject against even remote possibilities of injury, disability, or death.
8. The experiment should be conducted only by scientifically qualified persons. The highest degree of skill and care should be required through all stages of the experiment of those who conduct or engage in the experiment.
9. During the course of the experiment the human subject should be at liberty to bring the experiment to an end if he has reached the physical or mental state where continuation of the experiment seems to him to be impossible.
10. During the course of the experiment the scientist in charge must be prepared to terminate the experiment at any stage, if he has probably [sic] cause to believe, in the exercise of the good faith, superior skill and careful judgment required of him that a continuation of the experiment is likely to result in injury, disability, or death to the experimental subject.

From *Trials of war criminals before the Nuremberg military tribunals under control council law* 10(2):181-182, October 1946-April 1949.

| Box 10-9 | *The Declaration of Helsinki* |

INTRODUCTION

It is the mission of the physician to safeguard the health of the people. His or her knowledge and conscience are dedicated to the fulfillment of this mission.

The Declaration of Geneva of the World Medical Association binds the physician with the words, "The Health of my patient will be my first consideration," and the International Code of Medical Ethics declares that, "A physician shall act only in the patient's interest when providing medical care which might have the effect of weakening the physical and mental condition of the patient."

The purpose of biomedical research involving human subjects must be to improve diagnostic, therapeutic and prophylactic procedures and the understanding of the aetiology and pathogenesis of disease.

In current medical practice most diagnostic, therapeutic or prophylactic procedures involve hazards. This applies especially to biomedical research.

Medical progress is based on research which ultimately must rest in part on experimentation involving human subjects.

In the field of biomedical research a fundamental distinction must be recognized between medical research in which the aim is essentially diagnostic or therapeutic for a patient, and medical research, the essential object of which is purely scientific and without implying direct diagnostic or therapeutic value to the person subjected to the research.

Special caution must be exercised in the conduct of research which may affect the environment, and the welfare of animals used for research must be respected.

Because it is essential that the results of laboratory experiments be applied to human beings to further scientific knowledge and to help suffering humanity, the World Medical Association has prepared the following recommendations as a guide to every physician in biomedical research involving human subjects. They should be kept under review in the future. It must be stressed that the standards as drafted are only a guide to physicians all over the world. Physicians are not relieved from criminal, civil and ethical responsibilities under the laws of their own countries.

I. BASIC PRINCIPLES

1. Biomedical research involving human subjects must conform to generally accepted scientific principles and should be based on adequately performed laboratory and animal experimentation and on a thorough knowledge of the scientific literature.

2. The design and performance of each experimental procedure involving human subjects should be clearly formulated in an experimental protocol which should be transmitted for consideration, comment and guidance to a specially appointed committee independent of the investigator and the sponsor provided that this independent committee is in conformity with the laws and regulations of the country in which the research experiment is performed.

3. Biomedical research involving human subjects should be conducted only by scientifically qualified persons and under the supervision of a clinically competent medical person. The responsibility for the human subject must always rest with a medically qualified person and never rest on the subject of the research, even though the subject has given his or her consent.

4. Biomedical research involving human subjects cannot legitimately be carried out unless the importance of the objective is in proportion to the inherent risk to the subject.

5. Every biomedical research project involving human subjects should be preceded by careful assessment of predictable risks in comparison with foreseeable benefits to the subject or to others. Concern for the interests of the subject must always prevail over the interests of science and society.

Box 10-9	*The Declaration of Helsinki—cont'd*

I. BASIC PRINCIPLES—CONT'D

6. The right of the research subject to safeguard his or her integrity must always be respected. Every precaution should be taken to respect the privacy of the subject and to minimize the impact of the study on the subject's physical and mental integrity and on the personality of the subject.

7. Physicians should abstain from engaging in research projects involving human subjects unless they are satisfied that the hazards involved are believed to be predictable. Physicians should cease any investigation if the hazards are found to outweigh the potential benefits.

8. In publication of the results of his or her research, the physician is obliged to preserve the accuracy of the results. Reports of experimentation not in accordance with the principles laid down in this Declaration should not be accepted for publication.

9. In any research on human beings, each potential subject must be adequately informed of the aims, methods, anticipated benefits and potential hazards of the study and the discomfort it may entail. He or she should be informed that he or she is at liberty to abstain from participation in the study and that he or she is free to withdraw his or her consent to participation at any time. The physician should then obtain the subject's freely-given informed consent, preferably in writing.

10. When obtaining informed consent for the research project the physician should be particularly cautious if the subject is in a dependent relationship to him or her or may consent under duress. In that case the informed consent should be obtained by a physician who is not engaged in the investigation and who is completely independent of this official relationship.

11. In case of legal incompetence, informed consent should be obtained from the legal guardian in accordance with national legislation. Where physical or mental incapacity makes it impossible to obtain informed consent, or when the subject is a minor, permission from the responsible relative replaces that of the subject in accordance with national legislation.

    Whenever the minor child is in fact able to give a consent, the minor's consent must be obtained in addition to the consent of the minor's legal guardian.

12. The research protocol should always contain a statement of the ethical considerations involved and should indicate that the principles enunciated in the present Declaration are complied with.

II. MEDICAL RESEARCH COMBINED WITH PROFESSIONAL CARE (CLINICAL RESEARCH)

1. In the treatment of the sick person, the physician must be free to use a new diagnostic and therapeutic measure, if in his or her judgment it offers hope of saving life, reestablishing health or alleviating suffering.

2. The potential benefits, hazards and discomfort of a new method should be weighed against the advantages of the best current diagnostic and therapeutic methods.

3. In any medical study, every patient—including those of a control group, if any—should be assured of the best proven diagnostic and therapeutic method. This does not exclude the use of inert placebo in studies where no proven diagnostic or therapeutic method exists.

4. The refusal of the patient to participate in a study must never interfere with the physician-patient relationship.

5. If the physician considers it essential not to obtain informed consent, the specific reasons for this proposal should be stated in the experimental protocol for transmission to the independent committee (1, 2).

Continued

Box 10-9   *The Declaration of Helsinki—cont'd*

II. MEDICAL RESEARCH COMBINED WITH PROFESSIONAL CARE (CLINICAL RESEARCH)—cont'd

    6. The physician can combine medical research with professional care, the objective being the acquisition of new medical knowledge, only to the extent that medical research is justified by its potential diagnostic or therapeutic value for the patient.

III. NON-THERAPEUTIC BIOMEDICAL RESEARCH INVOLVING HUMAN SUBJECTS (NON-CLINICAL BIOMEDICAL RESEARCH)

    1. In the purely scientific application of medical research carried out on a human being, it is the duty of the physician to remain the protector of the life and health of that person on whom biomedical research is being carried out.

    2. The subjects should be volunteers—either healthy persons or patients for whom the experimental design is not related to the patient's illness.

    3. The investigator or the investigating team should discontinue the research if in his/her or their judgment it may, if continued, be harmful to the individual.

    4. In research on man, the interest of science and society should never take precedence over considerations related to the wellbeing of the subject.

From Committee on Medical Ethics, World Medical Association: Declaration of Helsinki. As amended by the 48th General Assembly, Somerset West, Republic of South Africa, October 1996.

In addition to complying with internationally accepted research codes of ethics, pharmacists must comply with federal regulations regarding the rights of research subjects. The federal regulations consist of the Department of Health and Human Services (DHHS) Code of Federal Regulations (CFR) Title 45A, part 46 and Title 21 of the Food and Drug Administration.[15] These regulations describe the composition and function of institutional review boards (IRBs), define the elements of informed consent, and provide the guidelines for documentation of informed consent.

The purpose of an IRB, also known as a *human research review board (HRRB)* or *human investigation committee (HIC)*, is to safeguard the rights and welfare of human research subjects. Investigators must submit all research protocols to the board and obtain approval before performing the research. Each institution in which human research is conducted must have this type of board. Noninstitution human research review boards are available for researchers engaged in clinical research outside specific institutions.[16]

The composition of research review boards is defined by law. Each board must be composed of at least five members with varying backgrounds capable of reviewing the types of research submitted to the board. Board membership also must be diverse. The board cannot be composed of all men, all women, or members of just one profession. At least one board member must be a nonscientist such as a lawyer, ethicist, or member of the clergy and at least one member must not otherwise be associated with the institution sponsoring the board.

Approval of research proposals is based on decisions regarding the relative risk to subjects, the way subjects are identified and selected, the way consent is obtained and documented, and the way subject confidentiality is maintained.

Research subjects must be informed to maintain the ethical principle of self-determination. Although the primary purpose of the board is to protect the rights of subjects, the board may comment on study design issues and the scientific merit of proposals.

A primary focus of the board is the content of the consent form and the way consent is obtained and documented. Written informed consent is required for most human research; consent for some relatively low-risk protocols may be obtained verbally. For consent to be valid, it must be voluntary. The written information must be in lay terms. Exculpatory language cannot be used and subjects must be considered legally competent. Federal regulations define required and additional elements of informed consent. Consent forms must contain specific elements; other elements are optional (Box 10-10).

Ethics and the Promotion of Prescription Drugs

Health professionals have begun to question the ethics of accepting gifts from drug companies.[17-19] Gifts range from low-cost items such as pens, notepads, clothing, textbooks, and meals to high-cost gifts such as all-expense-paid trips to luxury resorts and cash gifts. Pharmacists attending national pharmacy association meetings often attend industry-sponsored continuing education presentations, receptions, and parties and collect numerous trinkets from industry-sponsored exhibits.

The ethical issues are complex and evolve from the unique relationship between the pharmaceutical industry and health professionals. Unlike other types of advertising, pharmaceutical advertising targets health care professionals, who influence drug selection, and not patients, the ultimate consumers of the products. Pharmacists must acknowledge that ethical implications arise from accepting these gifts, no matter the monetary value of the gift.

The ethical implications of accepting gifts from the pharmaceutical industry involve issues of justness and obligations.[19] The cost of pharmaceutical gifts and other forms of advertising is included in the price of medications. Therefore some argue that spending patients' money without their knowledge or consent and without direct benefit is unjust. Gift giving also implies obligations on the part of the recipient. The obligations may be subtle, but even the appearance of an obligation may alter society's trust in the profession.

Guidelines regarding the relationships of health professionals with the pharmaceutical industry are evolving. Although most of the discussions have targeted physicians, the ethical issues and therefore the guidelines are applicable to other health professionals. The American Society of Hospital Pharmacists (ASHP) board of directors approved and published the ASHP guidelines on pharmacists' relationships with industry in 1992.[20] The guidelines address the issues of gifts and hospitality, continuing education, consultants and advisory arrangements, clinical research, and disclosure of information (Box 10-11).

Advance Directives

Advance directives are written legal documents that give a patient the ability to influence future treatment decisions if the patient loses the ability to make decisions. Advance directives are the focus of the Patient Self-Determination Act (PSDA), a law that went into effect on December 1, 1991.[21] The intent of the PSDA is to promote the knowledge and use of advance directives. The law, which applies to

---

Box 10-10 *Elements of Informed Consent*

REQUIRED ELEMENTS

1. A clear invitation (not a request or demand) to the individual to become a research subject
2. A statement that the study involves research and an explanation of the purposes of the research
3. A statement describing the reason the person was selected to participate in the study
4. The expected duration of the subject's participation in the study, a description of the procedures to be followed, and identification of experimental procedures
5. A description of reasonably foreseeable risks or discomforts to the subject
6. A statement on the availability of medical therapy and compensation for disability in case the subject is injured by participating in the study
7. A description of benefits to the subjects or others that may reasonably be expected from the research
8. A disclosure of alternatives to participating in the research study
9. A statement describing the extent to which confidentiality will be maintained and noting that the Food and Drug Administration may see the subject's records
10. An explanation of whom to contact for answers to questions about the research and subject's rights and whom to contact in the event a research-related injury occurs
11. A noncoercive disclaimer that participation is voluntary, refusal to participate involves no penalty or loss of benefits, and the subject may discontinue participation at any time without penalty or loss of benefits
12. A statement that the subject will receive a copy of the signed consent form
13. A place for signature and date of signature for the subject or legally authorized representative

OPTIONAL ELEMENTS

1. The approximate number of subjects in the study
2. The person or group conducting and funding the study
3. A statement that significant new findings relating to the subject's willingness to continue participation will be conveyed to the subject
4. A statement that the research may involve unforeseeable risks to the subject or fetus
5. A description of additional costs incurred by the patient participating in the study
6. A statement that the investigator may terminate the subject's participation with or without consent of the subject
7. A place for signature and date of signature for person obtaining consent and witness (if applicable)

Federal policy for the protection of human subjects: notes and rules, *Federal Register* 56:28002-28032, 1991.

all health care institutions (hospitals, nursing facilities, hospices, home care programs, and health maintenance organizations) that receive Medicare or Medicaid, requires institutions to give all individuals receiving medical care written information about their rights under state law to make decisions about their care, including the right to accept or refuse medical or surgical care. Individuals also must be given information about their rights to formulate advance directives. Institutions must prepare policies consistent with state law, document in each individual's medical record whether the individual has executed an advance directive, and develop public education programs.

The two main types of advance directives are living wills (Box 10-12) and du-

In the practice of their profession, pharmacists should be guided only by the consideration of patient care. Pharmacists should neither accept nor retain anything of value that has the potential to materially affect the ability to exercise judgments solely in the interest of patients. A useful criterion in determining acceptable activities and relationships is this: Would the pharmacist be willing to have these relationships generally known? Notwithstanding this responsibility, pharmacists may benefit from guidance in their relationships with industry. To this end, the following suggestions are offered.

GIFTS AND HOSPITALITY

Gifts, hospitality, or subsidies offered to pharmacists by industry should not be accepted if acceptance might influence or appear to others to influence the objectivity of clinical judgment or drug product selection and procurement.

CONTINUING EDUCATION

Providers of continuing education that accept industry funding for programs should develop and enforce policies to maintain complete control of program content.

Subsidies to underwrite the costs of continuing-education conferences, professional meetings, or staff development programs can contribute to the improvement of patient care and are permissible. Payments to defray the costs of a conference should not be accepted directly or indirectly from industry by pharmacists attending the conference or program. Contributions to special or educational funds for staff development are permissible as long as the selection of staff members who will receive the funds is made by the department of pharmacy.

It is appropriate for faculty at conferences or meetings to accept reasonable honoraria and to accept reimbursement for reasonable travel, lodging, and meal expenses. However, direct subsidies from industry should not be accepted to pay the costs of travel, lodging, or other personal expenses of pharmacists attending conferences or meetings, nor should subsidies be accepted to compensate for the pharmacist's time.

Scholarships or other special funds to permit pharmacy students, residents, and fellows to attend carefully selected educational conferences may be permissible as long as the selection of students, residents or fellows who will receive the funds is made by the academic or training institution.

CONSULTANTS AND ADVISORY ARRANGEMENTS

Consultants who provide genuine services for industry may receive reasonable compensation and accept reimbursement for travel, lodging, and meal expenses. Token consulting or advisory arrangements cannot be used to justify compensating pharmacists for their time, travel, lodging, and other out-of-pocket expenses.

CLINICAL RESEARCH

Pharmacists who participate in practice-based research of pharmaceuticals, devices, or other programs should conduct their activities in accord with basic precepts of accepted scientific methodology. Practice-based drug studies that are, in effect, promotional schemes to entice the use of a product or program are unacceptable.

DISCLOSURE OF INFORMATION

To avoid conflicts of interest or appearances of impropriety, pharmacists should disclose consultant/speaker arrangements or substantial personal financial holdings with companies under consideration for formulary inclusion or related decisions. To fully inform audiences, speakers and authors should disclose, when pertinent, consultant or speaker and research funding arrangements have been made with companies.

ADDITIONAL ISSUES

The advice in this document is nonexclusive and not intended to limit the legitimate exchange of prudent scientific information.

From ASHP guidelines on pharmacist's relationships with industry, *Am J Hosp Pharm* 49:154, 1992.

| Box 10-12 | *Example of a Living Will* |

To my Doctor:

While I have been at _____, I have discussed my wishes concerning my medical treatment in the event that I become extremely ill. I did this in the hope that if I made my wishes known beforehand, it would be easier for my doctors to know my preferences at a time when I am unable to express them.

If I become critically ill:

I want to be hospitalized.
I want to go into intensive care.
I want to have my heart revived if my heart stops.
I want to have surgery.
I want to be put on a breathing machine.

If I become terminally ill:

I want to be hospitalized.
I want my family members to decide whether I shall go into intensive care after they talk with my doctor.
I want my doctor to decide whether to revive me if my heart stops.
I want my family members to decide whether I shall have surgery after they talk with my doctor.
I want my family members to decide whether I shall be put on a breathing machine after they talk with my doctor.

If I am in an irreversible coma:

I want to be hospitalized.
I want my family members to decide whether I shall go into intensive care after they talk with my doctor.
I want my doctor to decide whether to revive me if my heart stops.

I want my family members to decide whether I shall have surgery after they talk with my doctor.
I do not want to be put on a breathing machine.
I want my family members to decide whether I shall be fed through a tube after they talk with my doctor.

If I am unable to make decisions for myself, I would like the following person to make necessary decisions on my behalf:

1. name (relationship)
   address

   phone: (home)
         (work)

If you cannot reach _____, I would like the following person to make the necessary decisions on my behalf:

2. name (relationship)
   address

   phone: (home)
         (work)

There will be a time when I want my doctor to stop keeping me alive.

I have provided this information in the hope that it will be easier to respect my wishes about my medical care at a time when I am unable to express them.

Patient _____ _____ _____
          name (printed)   (signature)   (date)

Witness _____ _____ _____
          name (printed)   (signature)   (date)

From Danis M et al: A prospective study of advance directives for life-sustaining care, *N Engl J Med* 324:8882, 1991.

rable powers of attorney (Box 10-13); some hybrid documents combine elements of each document. A living will provides direction regarding specific medical treatments the person does or does not want at the end of life and can serve as a general reference for decision making. The advantage of living wills is that individuals can identify specific interventions such as surgery, dialysis, chest compression, in-

Box 10-13 *Example of a Durable Power of Attorney*

I. _____. residing   at
                     (principal—print your name)

_____
      (street)   (city or town)   (state)

appoint as my Health Care Agent _____
                                     (name of person you choose as agent)

of _____
    (street)   (city or town)   (state)   (phone)

    Optional: If my agent is unwilling or unable to serve, then I appoint as my alternate

_____
               (name of person you choose as alternate)

of _____.
    (street)   (city or town)   (state)   (phone)

    My agent shall have the authority to make all health care decisions for me, subject to any limitations I state below, if I am unable to make decisions myself. My agent's authority becomes effective if my attending physician determines in writing that I lack the capacity to make or to communicate health care decisions. My agent is then to have the same authority to make health care decisions as I would if I had the capacity to make them, *except* (here list the limitations, *if any,* you wish to place on your agent's authority):

    I direct my agent to make decisions on the basis of my agent's assessment of my personal wishes. If my personal wishes are unknown, my agent is to make decisions on the basis of my agent's assessment of my best interests. Photocopies of this Health Care Proxy shall have the same force and effect as the original.

Signed _____

    Complete only if principal is physically unable to sign: I have signed the principal's name above at his or her direction in the presence of the principal and two witnesses.

_____
                         (name)

_____
                        (street)

_____
           (city or town)   (state)

Witness Statement

    We, the undersigned, each witnessed the signing of this Health Care Proxy by the principal or at the direction of the principal and state that the principal appears to be at least 18 years of age, of sound mind, and under no constraint or undue influence. Neither of us is named as the health care agent or alternate in this document.

In our presence this _____ day of _____ 199_____.

Witness 1 _____   Witness 2_____
              (signature)   (signature)
Name (print) _____   Name (print)_____

Address _____   Address_____

_____   _____

From Annas GJ: The health care proxy and the living will, *N Engl J Med* 324:1210-1213, 1991.

tubation and mechanical ventilation they do not want. Living wills are especially useful for patients with chronic illnesses. However, living wills require that individuals predict future acceptable and unacceptable medical interventions, often without an accurate or complete understanding of all available options or the implications of each option. Living wills do not appoint an alternate decision maker and often must be interpreted when tough decisions have to be made regarding end-of-life treatment decisions. Written durable powers of attorney appoint an alternate decision maker (the proxy) who is legally empowered to make decisions regarding the care of the patient. A durable power of attorney is activated whenever the patient is incapacitated. The advantage of the durable power of attorney is that an individual can identify a person to engage in future discussions regarding specific clinical situations. However, the durable power of attorney does not by itself tell the proxy the decisions to make on the patient's behalf. The scope of proxy responsibilities varies by state statute but generally empowers the proxy to admit the person to an acute or chronic care facility and arrange for and consent to medical and surgical treatment.

One of the most common problems associated with advance directives is that the document may not be available when decisions have to be made. The document may be locked in a safe deposit box, filed in a lawyer's office, or held by distant offspring. Another problem is that the document may be out of date and not accurately reflect the patient's desires as the patient faces the realities of end-of-life illnesses and gains experience with available technology and other interventions. Pharmacists should be aware of the presence of advance directives and ensure that therapeutic decisions are made in accordance with the patient's wishes.

Withholding and Withdrawing Medical Interventions

The issues of withholding and withdrawing medical interventions are relatively recent ethical dilemmas. *Withholding of life support* and *withdrawal of life support* refer to decisions to withhold or withdraw medical interventions with the expectation that the patient will die from the change in support.[24] Technologic and pharmaceutical advances provide health care professionals with effective tools for prolonging life. At issue, however, is the quality of life and the right of patients to make their own decisions. Competent patients or alternate decision makers have the right to choose. Health care professionals have the ethical responsibility to inform patients and alternate decision makers of choices and honor their decisions. Although the responsibility for withholding or withdrawing life support rests with the patient or proxy and the patient's physician, broad consensus is sought among all health professionals involved in the care of the patient. Every effort is made to honor the patient's wishes regarding these difficult decisions.

SELF-ASSESSMENT QUESTIONS

1 Which of the following is the fundamental moral principle on which all ethical behavior is based?
   a. Do good and avoid evil
   b. Do what is best for society as a whole
   c. Obey all federal laws
   d. Maintain patient confidentiality
   e. Obey all state laws

2 What do the pharmacy, nursing, and medical codes of ethics have in common?
   a. Hippocrates wrote all three codes.
   b. All three contain issue-specific guidelines.
   c. All three are based on the Declaration of Helsinki.
   d. All three were written in the sixth century BC.
   e. All three provide broad-based directives.

3 The patient's bill of rights was created to do which of the following?
   a. Protect institutions from lawsuits
   b. Advise hospitalized patients of their rights
   c. Prevent patients from making bad decisions
   d. Give autonomy to alternate decision makers
   e. Advise ambulatory patients of their rights

4 According to the patient's bill of rights, patients have the right to do which of the following?
   a. Receive considerate and respectful care
   b. Refuse a recommended treatment plan
   c. Review records pertaining to their medical care
   d. All of the above
   e. None of the above

5 Which of the following actions violate patient confidentiality?
   a. Discussing a patient case in a public elevator
   b. Disclosing the results of diagnostic tests to friends of the patient
   c. Allowing public access to electronically stored patient information
   d. All of the above
   e. A and C above

6 What is wrong with a research review board composed of four male physicians?
   a. A board must have at least five members.
   b. More than one type of profession must be represented.
   c. Both men and women must be members.
   d. All of the above
   e. None of the above

7 The primary purpose of an institutional review board is to do which of the following?
   a. Judge the scientific merit of proposed research
   b. Locate funding sources for proposed research
   c. Safeguard the rights and welfare of human subjects
   d. Analyze the results of studies
   e. Protect the rights of researchers

8 Which one of the following is an optional element of informed consent?
   a. A description of additional costs to the subject
   b. A description of reasonably foreseeable risks
   c. A disclosure of alternatives to participation in the study
   d. A clear invitation to become a research subject
   e. A place for the signature of the subject

9 According to the ASHP guidelines on pharmacists' relationships with industry, which of the following is inappropriate?
   a. Accepting money to pay for personal expenses arising from attending a conference

b. Accepting a reasonable honorarium for work performed
c. Participating in practice-based drug studies that are in fact promotional schemes
d. All of the above
e. A and C above

10 Which one of the following statements regarding living wills is FALSE?
a. Living wills provide specific information regarding medical treatment the patient does or does not want to have at the end of life.
b. Living wills often must be interpreted.
c. Living wills appoint a proxy.
d. Living wills may become outdated.
e. Living wills provide patients with the means to influence future treatment decisions.

REFERENCES

1. Tempkin O, Temkin CL: *Ancient medicine: selected papers of Ludwig Edelstein,* Baltimore, 1967, Johns Hopkins University.
2. Knoepfler JF: Eidesformein für Arzt, Apotheker Hebammen, Wundarzt und Frauenwirt zu Amberg, *Arch Gesch Med* 11:318, 1919.
3. A code of ethics adopted by the Philadelphia College of Pharmacy, *Am J Pharm* 20:148-151, 1848.
4. *Code of ethics for pharmacists,* Washington, DC, 1995, American Pharmaceutical Association.
5. Vottero LD: The code of ethics for pharmacists, *Am J Health-Syst Pharm* 21:2096, 1995.
6. *Oath of a pharmacist,* Alexandria, VA, 1995, American Association of Colleges of Pharmacy.
7. King LS: IX. The AMA gets a new code of ethics, *JAMA* 249:1338-1342, 1983.
8. American Medical Association Council on Ethical and Judicial Affairs: *Current opinions of the Council on Ethical and Judicial Affairs of the American Medical Association,* Chicago, 1992, American Medical Association.
9. Kelly C: *Dimensions of professional nursing,* New York, 1962, Macmillan.
10. American Nurses Association: *Code for nurses and interpretive statements,* Kansas City, MO, 1985, American Nurses Association.
11. *The patient's bill of rights,* Chicago, 1992, American Hospital Association.
12. Rothman DJ: Ethics and human experimentation, *N Engl J Med* 317:1195-1199, 1987.
13. *Trials of war criminals before the Nuremberg military tribunals under control council law* 10(2):181-182, October 1946-April 1949.
14. Committee on Medical Ethics, World Medical Association: Declaration of Helsinki. As amended by the 48th General Assembly, Somerset West, Republic of South Africa, October 1996.
15. Federal policy for the protection of human subjects: notes and rules, *Federal Register* 56:28002-28032, 1991.
16. Herman SS: A noninstitutional review board comes of age, *IRB* 11:1-6, 1989.
17. Zoloth AM: The need for ethical guidelines for relationships between pharmacists and the pharmaceutical industry, *Am J Hosp Pharm* 48:551-552, 1991.
18. Goldfinger SE: Physicians and the pharmaceutical industry, *Ann Intern Med* 112:624-626, 1990.
19. Chren M-M, Landefeld S, Murray TH: Doctors, drug companies, and gifts, *JAMA* 262:3448-3451, 1989.
20. ASHP guidelines on pharmacists' relationships with industry, *Am J Hosp Pharm* 49:154, 1992.

21. *Consolidated omnibus budget reconciliation act of 1990,* Pub. Law No. 101-508, Paragraphs 4206, 4751.
22. Danis M et al: A prospective study of advance directives for life-sustaining care, *N Engl J Med* 324:882-888, 1991.
23. Annas GJ: The health care proxy and the living will, *N Engl J Med* 324:1210-1213, 1991.
24. Smedira NG et al: Withholding and withdrawal of life support from the critically ill, *N Engl J Med* 322:309-315, 1990.

Answer Key for Self-Assessment Questions

Chapter 1
1 e
2 d
3 b
4 a
5 d
6 c
7 c
8 b
9 d
10 d

Chapter 2
1 d
2 b
3 d
4 e
5 a
6 c
7 c
8 e
9 a
10 d

Chapter 3
1 c
2 d
3 e
4 d
5 b
6 d
7 a
8 d
9 a
10 b

Chapter 4
1 e
2 c
3 d
4 b
5 d
6 e
7 a
8 c
9 c
10 b

Chapter 5
1 d
2 b
3 a
4 c
5 e
6 b
7 a
8 c
9 d
10 e

Chapter 6
1 b
2 a
3 d
4 b
5 d
6 c
7 b
8 a
9 d
10 a

Chapter 7
1 e
2 c
3 d
4 c
5 b
6 a
7 a

8 c
9 e
10 a

Chapter 8
1 e
2 c
3 b
4 c
5 a
6 d
7 a
8 c
9 b
10 d

Chapter 9
1 d
2 a
3 d
4 a
5 b
6 c
7 d
8 d
9 c
10 d

Chapter 10
1 a
2 e
3 b
4 d
5 d
6 d
7 c
8 a
9 e
10 c

Index

A

Abdominal examination, 79-82
Abdominal reflex, 86
Abducens nerve, 84
ABO blood typing, 104
Abuse
  drug, 44-45
  substance, 131
Accommodation, pupillary, 66
Achilles reflex, 86
Acid-fast stain, 112
Acoustic nerve, 85
Active listening, 18
Acuity, visual, 66
Admitting resident, 10
Adrenal hormones, 98
Adrenal tests, 97
Adrenocorticotropic hormone, 99
Advance directive, 203, 206
Adverse drug reaction, 178
  medication history and, 47
Air conduction, 65
Alanine aminotransferase, 102
Albumin, 100-101, 114
Alcohol use, 131
Alkaline phosphatase, 100
Allergy, 47
Allied health care professional, 6
Alpha-fetoprotein, 102
Ambulatory electrocardiography, 96
American Hospital Association,
      196-197
American Hospital Formulary Service, 179
American Pharmaceutical Association,
      193
American Society of Health-System
      Pharmacists, 4-5
American Society of Hospital
      Pharmacists, 203, 205
Ammonia, 100
Amylase, 97
Anergy panel, 112

Angiography, 93, 95
Antagonistic patient, 30
Anthropometrics, 115-116
Antibody, 109-110
Anti-DNA antibody, 110
Antigen, carcinoembryonic, 102
Antinuclear antibody, 109-110
Anus, 82
Aperture, ophthalmoscope, 62
Arterial blood gas, 116-117, 120
Artery, retinal, 67
Article, journal, 180-181
Ascites, 81
Aspartate aminotransferase, 102
Aspiration, bone marrow, 109
Assessment, physical, 56-91
  abbreviations used in, 57-58
  abdominal, 79-82
  cardiovascular, 72-79
  chest and lungs, 69-72
  communication and, 19
  equipment for, 59-61
  genitourinary, 82-83
  head and neck, 64-69
  musculoskeletal, 83
  neurologic, 83-90
  process of, 56, 58
  skin, 62-64
  technique of, 58-59
Assistant, physician, 8
Attending physician, 9
Attending rounds, 11
Audiovisual materials, 35
Auscultation
  abdominal, 80
  cardiovascular assessment and, 75-76
  respiratory system assessment and,
      71
Autoantibody
  organ-specific, 111
  types of, 109-110
Axilla, 79

Notes

Notes

Notes

Notes

Notes

Notes

Notes

Notes

Notes

Notes